THE

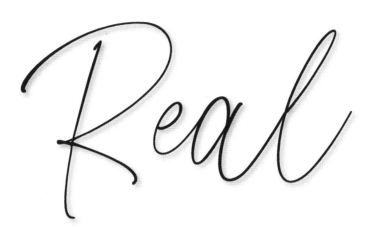

MEDITERRANEAN DIET

A practical guide to understanding and achieving the healthiest diet in the world

ISBN 10: 1903-500-57-5
ISBN 13: 978-1903-500-57-6

Printed and bound in the United Kingdom by 4edge Ltd, 22 Eldon Way Industrial Estate, Hockley, Essex, SS5 4AD.

Back cover image Courtesy of Boundary Bend, Australia

Simon, in his enchanting, sustainable and constantly regenerating wit, has delivered an easy-to-enjoy, digest and benefit from (no pun intended) book. Read this book alone or with friends, and draw from his rich knowledge and experience. With plentiful, diverse but never overbearing scientific evidence, Simon manages to creatively blend a story that opens the door to the amazing, mythical and thousands years-old Mediterranean way of eating. He has cracked open the kitchen door for you to explore and immerse yourself into this nutritious lifestyle. So why are you still standing there? Come on in...let your imagination lead the way.
– Dr Tassos Kyriakides PhD, Yale School of Public Health

The Mediterranean Diet stands out in nutrition science research as one of the healthiest dietary patterns in the world and Dr Simon Poole has captured its elements, history, science and deliciousness in this fabulous book. With extra virgin olive oil at its heart, this pattern of eating not only makes everything taste better, it also reduces the risk of many chronic diseases, puts the brake on ageing and is good for the body from the gut to the brain and everything in between. This book gives you the know-how to put it into practise no matter where you are in the world.
– Dr Joanna McMillan PhD, Nutrition scientist, Dietitian &
Fellow Lifestyle Medicine

Dr Simon Poole has written an excellent book on what quite possibly could be the best diet in the world that could save lives and the planet. Eat up!"
– Dr Rupy Aujla, MBBS, MRCGP. Founder, "The Doctor's Kitchen"

I was impressed with this well-written and comprehensive account of the health benefits of the Mediterranean diet, together with a good and readable summary of the science behind the diet. It includes many relevant and useful food facts and is rounded off with a series of truly delicious recipes from chefs from around the Mediterranean and beyond.
– Richard, Lord Balfe, Past Honorary President of the British Dietetic Association and NNEdPro Global Centre for Nutrition and Health

Table of Contents

Foreword

I never dreamed that a visit to West London organised by the Guild of Food Writers for what was billed as an Olive Oil Tasting would prove to be such a life-changing and enhancing experience for me.

We were addressed by Dr Simon Poole on the health-giving properties of Extra Virgin Olive Oil and the Mediterranean Diet. I was fascinated by what he had to say and asked for a copy of his presentation after he had finished, which he kindly sent me.

I have used Extra Virgin Olive Oil ever since, instead of any other oils, and experienced health benefits as a result; in common with many men in their seventies I was on statins, something I have been able to cease taking, and had been diagnosed as pre-diabetic, now no longer a problem.

Early in 2020, I had a full medical, and that produced the best results that I have ever achieved in recent years in terms of cholesterol level, blood pressure and blood sugar, which I was delighted about.

I have become a complete convert and even take Extra Virgin Olive Oil with me when I am travelling, and I have sent his presentation to a number of my friends.

The time-honoured adage 'you are what you eat' is so true, and I would like to recommend that you follow his advice and reap the health benefits.

– The Rt Hon Richard Bridgeman, The Earl of Bradford

About the Author

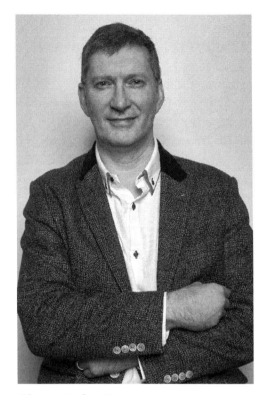

Photo: Pedro Rus

Dr Simon Poole is a family physician, author, broadcaster and an acclaimed international authority on the Mediterranean Diet. Simon is based in Cambridge, United Kingdom and has been involved in research and teaching with the University of Cambridge. He has been a member of the British Medical Association Public Health Committee and was awarded Fellowship of the Association in 2019 for services to the BMA.

He is a Senior International Collaborator with the Cambridge Global Centre for Nutrition and Health and a founding Scientific Advisory Board Member of the Olive Wellness Institute. Simon has regularly published on the subject of nutrition, lifestyle and public health in the press and scientific journals including *Nutrition and Food Science* and the *International Journal of Clinical Practice*.

He has presented on national and international radio and television, including the BBC programme *Nadiya's Family Favourites*. Conference addresses have included presentations at institutions such as the National Association of Primary Care, the Royal College of General Practitioners, the International Congress of the European Society of Cardiology, the Italian Trade Commission, the Fine Food Fair at OIympia, the Institute of Health Sciences of the USA and the Boston Common Ground Convention.

Simon was co-organiser and chair, in association with the University of Florence, of the Food Values conference series at the Vatican Pontifical Academy of Sciences. He is a regular guest lecturer for Viking Ocean Cruises. Simon has taught at the London Olive Oil Times Sommelier course, the London International Olive Oil Competition and presented at the North American Olive Oil Association Conference, as well as the World Olive Oil Exhibition in Madrid, the World Olive Health Awards in Malaga and the Old Parliament in Athens, receiving special commendation awards for contribution to the promotion of the Mediterranean Diet and communication of the health benefits to the public.

His first book *The Olive Oil Diet* was published in 2016. Co-authored with Judy Ridgway, the *Olive Oil Diet* was awarded the International Gourmand Prize for the World's Best Mediterranean Cuisine Book and was named the National Best Diet Book. To date it has been translated into Spanish, Turkish and Bulgarian.

Acknowledgements

I would like to thank all those you have encouraged and inspired me to write this book, to advance the understanding and dissemination of the Mediterranean Diet. The evidence for the many benefits of the Mediterranean Diet is well established, widely accepted and based on many thousands of peer reviewed published papers from researchers who dedicate their careers to nutritional science. This book has been written with the intention of bringing together that current knowledge in a concise way and therefore references to specific studies are not included.

I am deeply indebted to my sister Penny for fastidiously editing the text to ensure it can be understood by a non-scientific audience, and to Associate Professor Daniela Martini, Department of Nutrition, Milan University for critiquing the accurate representation of the science for a general readership.

I am grateful for the support and patience of my wife Roslyn and to my publishers Cambridge Academic for recognising the need for a book describing the extraordinary "secrets and alchemy" of the Mediterranean Diet, the understanding of which I have witnessed to have the power to change lives.

Disclaimer

Information included in this book reflects interpretation of current evidence based on peer reviewed publications in scientific literature. The advice is based on this evidence, involving population observational and controlled trials of adult populations. It should not replace the guidance of prescribed medication of a personal physician and in the event of allergies or special prescribed diets, further medical direction should be sought. Reference to this information should be made as an indication to make positive changes in diet and lifestyle. Regular exercise is also important to maintain a good state of health. If any individual has concerns about their need or capacity to make lifestyle changes, they should seek further medical advice.

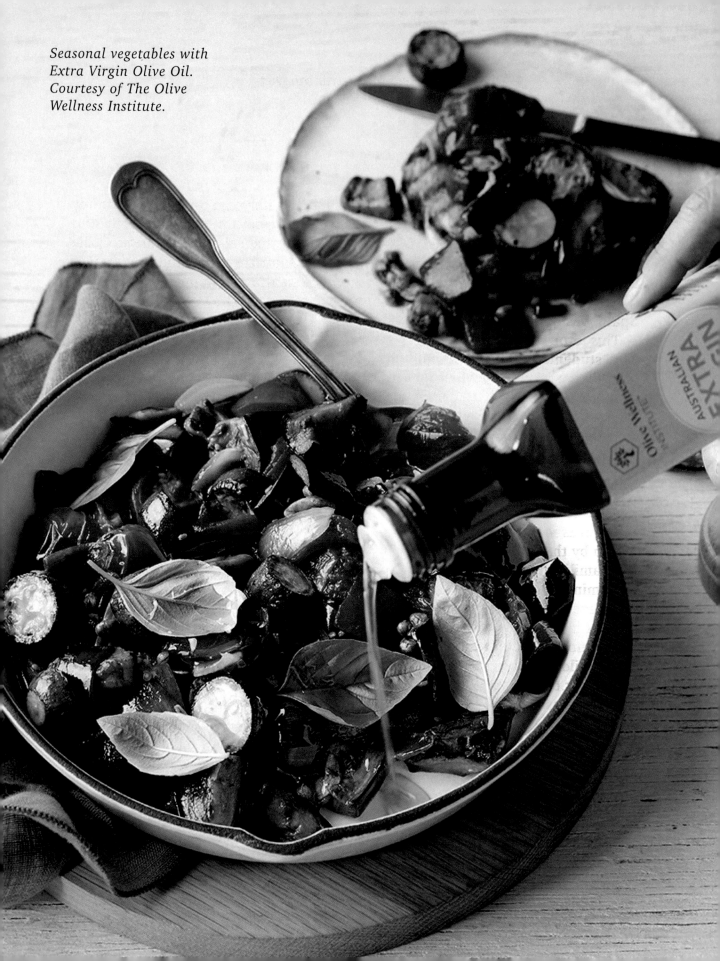

Seasonal vegetables with Extra Virgin Olive Oil. Courtesy of The Olive Wellness Institute.

Preface

My journey to discover the secrets of the real Mediterranean Diet began in my consulting rooms in Cambridge over twenty years ago. I picked up a copy of a respected medical journal and started to read a statistical analysis showing the rates of chronic diseases such as heart disease, stroke, dementia and cancer amongst different European populations. The health and longevity of people living on the shores of a Greek island or amongst the olive groves of central Spain was quite extraordinary.

This brought back vivid memories of experiences travelling in the region as a student. I recalled leaning against my backpack on a dusty country road somewhere in central Anatolia waiting for a bus and meeting a stranger who, with a combination of broken English and hand gestures, made it clear that I was invited to a wedding in his mountain village. I shall never forget the enthusiastic welcome and warm hospitality shown to me that day. I remember the barber insisting on bestowing the closest shave of my life and hearing the hauntingly beautiful music of the oud and other traditional instruments as the women and men of the village gathered at either end of the square to begin the festivities.

Most of all I recollect the food. Set on long trestle tables as the sun set over the Taurus mountains, the colourful array of dishes created with skill, love and gossip by the ladies of the village was far removed from the foods with which I was familiar. There were tomatoes baked with herbs, purple skinned aubergines swimming in fresh green olive oil, countless other *meze* dishes with flatbreads and huge clay pots of simmering chicken and bean stew. The aromas and flavours were as memorable as the atmosphere of hospitality, conviviality and celebration. As the elders of the community watched their children, grandchildren and great grandchildren dancing I understood that old age was not something to be feared, but rather to be embraced and enjoyed.

My interest increased over time as scientific research began to reveal just how powerful this diet can be. I began to tell the stories of the Mediterranean Diet to patients and colleagues, with a particular focus on how best to support others to discover and share the extraordinary benefits of this way of life. For some there have been moments of epiphany, when an understanding of the way the diet works has sparked profound changes in their life which can be measured in their improved health and wellbeing. Others simply adopt the Mediterranean Diet because it is such a pleasurable way to enjoy truly wholesome foods and to celebrate the art of preparing and sharing simple, yet exquisite meals. In my experience it is the understanding and enjoyment of the Mediterranean Diet which results in an enduring love affair with the lifestyle.

I have been very fortunate to have been invited to speak at conferences in recent years and have had the privilege to meet many dedicated ambassadors for the Mediterranean Diet from different backgrounds. I have found that everyone has a story to tell of how their relationship with the Mediterranean Diet began. It has been fascinating to meet leading scientists in the field, some of whom specialise in the most detailed biochemistry of nutrition, and to attend conferences in hallowed venues such as the Vatican's Pontifical Academy of Sciences and the Harvard Club in New York. The understanding of the science of the Mediterranean Diet is advancing rapidly and has the potential, if more widely known, to profoundly change our lives.

It has been just as enlightening meeting the farmer who stoops to pick up a handful of the Andalusian soil which he testifies with passion provides the distinctive taste of his local vegetables. I have learned how a cheese is crafted with unique moulds in cool caves in the hills of Tuscany, and how generations of custodians of an ancient olive grove in Sparta have carefully managed the balanced ecosystem to produce an Extra Virgin Olive Oil which has won awards in London and Tokyo. I have witnessed the concerns in once-fertile lands experiencing unprecedented drought, and seen the Saharan sands swept northwards by winds which threaten to stifle the annual crop pollination. I have had the joy of hand harvesting an ancient olive tree amongst Roman ruins under the warmth of a Tunisian sun and being teased for failing to keep pace with the skilled women and men of the town. Chefs, from the streets of Manhattan to the Australian Outback have shown how the traditional dishes of the Mediterranean can be transformed into works of culinary art whilst maintaining the link to the simplicity of their origins.

There is so much we can learn from those who study or practise the Mediterranean Diet. Some of that knowledge is published and some is intuitive or passed from generation to generation. Scientific findings are recorded in research journals, whilst its broader wisdom is taught by grandmothers in the kitchens of houses in small villages and by farmers to sons and daughters in the field. Finally, there are some physicians beginning to teach it to patients and students and a few enlightened regional governments are initiating programmes to help children to understand and benefit from learning how to enjoy the preparation and consumption of the healthy foods of the Mediterranean Diet.

So many chronic diseases, including cancers, heart disease, stroke, diabetes, dementia and many other conditions can often be prevented with the adoption of a healthier lifestyle, especially with a change in diet. Chronic diseases have the potential to cause suffering for individuals and their loved ones over many years, often leading to early death. We have also seen that such conditions can make people more susceptible to be hit hardest by new and devastating infections. Our nutritional state can have a significant effect on our immune system. Malnutrition is now a description not limited to an inadequacy of supply of food, but more commonly refers to the effects of a poor-quality diet including its central role in the exponential rise in obesity and diabetes. The time to understand and achieve a truly healthy diet is now.

As a physician an important part of my role is to communicate messages of health clearly and succinctly to make a difference in our busy lives. My job is to translate the complexities of the science of health into ideas which can be easily understood and enable the creation of manageable, achievable, and rewarding positive changes. Some time ago, as it became apparent that the majority of chronic illnesses might be prevented through lifestyle changes, I began to advise my patients in Cambridge to adopt a more Mediterranean way of eating.

Many were astonished at improvements in their blood pressure, cholesterol levels, weight and even their sense of happiness and wellbeing. They reported feeling fitter and more energetic. But what became clear was that although it was easy to give general lifestyle advice, it was impossible to fully explain the Mediterranean Diet in a short consultation. I now spend much of my time speaking to different audiences on the subject of the Mediterranean Diet. They tell me that they simply did not know what they did not know. I was recently asked if it would be possible to write a short and easy guide to reveal the treasures of the diet. This book is written with the aim of explaining the Mediterranean Diet in a way which tells the story of the extraordinary discoveries of how it really works. Its ambition is to change lives – to dramatically and permanently make a difference to our health and enjoyment of life.

This book is dedicated to all those who have devoted their lives to sharing their knowledge and passion for the Mediterranean Diet, in particular those whom I have met on my travels who have been so hospitable and generous. In gathering together an appreciation of the Mediterranean Diet for a wider audience, it is my hope that I may in some small way honour those many acts of kindness.

Introduction

We hear a lot about the Mediterranean Diet. We read about it in newspapers, magazines and there are glossy books full of recipes on the subject. It is commonly described as the "gold standard diet" for our generation and it is recommended by doctors, governments and the World Health Organisation. It wins accolades year after year in head-to-head comparisons of sustainable healthy diets, including being the undisputed *US News* Best Diet champion for a number of years.

Respected journals have published articles which estimate that if we moved to a similar dietary pattern as many as 20,000 deaths could be prevented annually in the United Kingdom and staggering potential savings in healthcare costs could be achieved. For example, with just a twenty percent increase in adoption of a Mediterranean style diet an estimated annual saving of eight billion dollars could be made to the costs of heart disease alone in the USA. This rises to an annual saving of more than thirty billion dollars if adherence to the diet increased by eighty percent from current levels.

If the power of the Mediterranean Diet could be put in a pill, the pharmaceutical industry would have done so years ago, and all of us surely would be taking it.

The status of the Mediterranean Diet is based on a substantial sum of evidence showing that following the diet reduces the risk of a broad range of chronic diseases. It is associated with significantly more healthy years of living and can contribute to much better mental health and wellbeing. It is a diet for life, and a lifestyle for the body and mind.

There really need be no arguments about the basics of what we eat. There is no place for the latest celebrity diet fad or the loudest quarrel on social media about which food to demonise next. Reducing processed products, enjoying real, natural food and knowing which ingredients are on the plate will result in better health. There is one diet, however, that has emerged to top the charts and which has the proof to back up claims that it can add even more quantity of years to life and quality of life to years.

The evidence has gathered pace over decades. Sometimes the results from a large study create a leap forward in our appreciation of the extent to which the Mediterranean Diet exerts its life-changing effects, and occasionally this comes to public view in newspapers and magazines. More often it is the many smaller steps which come from research published by laboratories across the world which provide even greater insight into how and why the diet works.

Some of the more nuanced conclusions from these analyses show us the importance of food production, how ingredients may interact in a meal and how the trillions of bacteria which reside in our gut can have a dramatic effect on the outcome of our dietary choices.

Yet little attention is paid to these details when it comes to recommendations from even the most trusted sources of information. This is perhaps because those advising us may not wish to complicate the simple message to eat more fruit and vegetables. Governments and reliable authorities on health focus on the most basic principles. Following this advice, and even applying the fundamentals of what is commonly characterised as a "Mediterranean style diet" may lift a person's diet from a "bad diet" to one that is perhaps above mediocre or even to what might be said to be a "good diet".

But to access the true power of the real Mediterranean Diet we need to understand what constitutes excellence in the diet in a way that is not achieved by most articles or books on the subject – not least because it is the happiest of coincidences that with the realisation of excellence comes the greatest enjoyment and taste.

The Mediterranean Diet has its origins in the traditions of ancient civilizations. The philosophers of those cultures first described the importance of appreciating an idea in terms of answering questions about "who, what, why, where, when, how and with what". The Mediterranean Diet can create health and pleasure for those who understand what it is and why it works. The principles of the Mediterranean Diet can be applied anywhere in the world and its beneficial effects are measurable immediately and at any age. When people adopt this pattern of eating the effects can be quickly appreciated. Final chapters of this book provide a practical and easy-to-follow guide of how to apply the principles of the Mediterranean Diet and with what key ingredients to achieve transformation in just 7 days. The idea of the real Mediterranean Diet will be truly explored and revealed.

Getting to Know the Mediterranean Diet – Asking the Right Questions

How much do we really know about the diet and how to bring it to our busy daily lives? On the face of it there is simplicity in the principles of the Mediterranean Diet and it is often described in a sentence or two. It does not contain highly-processed "convenience" foods, involves the preparation of meals with healthy ingredients and is low in refined sugars and unhealthy fats. When it comes to the foods of the Mediterranean Diet, we are generally told that it means eating more vegetables, fruits, wholegrains, fish, legumes and olive oil whilst cutting down on our red meat and dairy intake.

But is this the whole story? Does it truly reflect in a few words the secret to a long and healthy life? Is there a risk that we might be missing some of the essential characteristics of the diet?

Most discussions about diet these days focus on the big three macronutrients – carbohydrates, fats and proteins. In the simplest terms these macronutrients in foods provide energy and the building blocks for life and constitute the largest nutrient groups in terms of the volume we eat. There have been promoters of a "low fat Mediterranean Diet" and we now read about "the low carb Mediterranean Diet". Is this misappropriation, misuse or even abuse of the Mediterranean Diet? The Mediterranean Diet is in fact neither low in fat or in carbohydrates as a proportion of calorie intake. Its effects are actually much more interesting and exciting than that, and probably relate more to enjoying the beneficial constituents rather than reducing the negative ones. The impact of the diet is through what might be termed "positive nutrition". This is a far cry from an ethos of avoiding particular food groups, and a rather better place to be.

The advantages of the Mediterranean Diet are based on the particular subtypes of macronutrients and also on micronutrients such as vitamins and minerals found in smaller quantities in foods. Other compounds which confer health from plants are called phytonutrients (phyto meaning "from a plant"), or bioactive compounds, acknowledging their influence on our state of health. For those who like to use the purest definition of a nutrient – a substance required for survival and growth – these extraordinarily powerful chemicals may not even be permitted to be described as nutrients, yet they are extraordinarily important. Clearly, when it comes to nutrients and health, size and definition is not everything.

Is the Mediterranean Diet just a list of ingredients, or is the way food is prepared, cooked and combined together crucial factors in its success? Do nutrients act synergistically and if so, how and with what effects?

Is the Mediterranean Diet really low in dairy products? In Greece and Southern France in particular, the intake of cheese and yoghurt is actually rather high. What about the sugars in fruits? Should we now have reason to fear them? And what do we mean by olive oil? Does it need to be Extra Virgin Olive Oil?

It turns out that questions such as these are really rather fundamental.

In Search of the Real Mediterranean Diet

Probably the most important key to unlocking the health of the Mediterranean Diet is in understanding Extra Virgin Olive Oil, the beneficial power of which we now understand to be largely driven by compounds known as polyphenols. These bioactive phytochemicals are present in plant foods and are especially rich in the Mediterranean Diet. They are a compelling illustration that the focus of dietary advice should not be on macronutrients alone. Polyphenols have unique and extraordinary anti-inflammatory, antioxidant and healing properties. This is exciting the world of science, yet how many people are aware of their existence or know how to recognise them in the taste of an Extra Virgin Olive Oil and other ingredients of the Mediterranean Diet? What is it about foods such as broccoli, kale, onions, green tea, blueberries and tomatoes or more exotic produce like pomegranates, dates, or rosemary and turmeric that has given them "superfood" status in popular nutritional stories? Are polyphenols the common feature and can these compounds be seen in their colour and experienced in their aromas and tastes?

Of course, if we all were to eat more freshly prepared ingredients and reduce our consumption of "junk food" we would be healthier, and for many this is the limit of their understanding of the Mediterranean Diet. To uncover the truly extraordinary revelations of the power of the diet however we need to dig a little deeper. There are lengthy scientific textbooks dedicated to the subject, but we do not need a degree in nutritional science to understand the secrets in a traditional kitchen on a Greek island or in a Spanish tapas bar. Whilst it is important to remain faithful to original and sometimes complicated science, telling the stories in a straightforward way is essential. When we have understanding, we are much more empowered to make the right decisions and choices.

The Theory of Everything

The aim of this book is to describe the benefits of the Mediterranean Diet in an historic and modern context, to explore the root cause of chronic diseases and to consider the important ingredients in a diet which can reduce and reverse these processes. Science is finally getting to a place where there is a much clearer understanding of the common causes of disease. Rather than trying to explain how the chemistry of nutrition might fit together, it is wiser to take the observed power of the Mediterranean Diet, and to drill down why it works; to deconstruct and understand each of the layers of its effects. This is the way to unravel the nutritional equivalent of the "theory of everything". On the journey of "joining the dots" to create the full picture of the Mediterranean Diet and how it works there are some fascinating points of interest, including discoveries about the ways in which foods interact for health when combined together, learning about individual ingredients and their effect on our gut microbes and genes, as well as the role of bioactive compounds such as polyphenols abundant in colourful plants. Only when these fundamental aspects of nutrition are understood is it possible to get the most enjoyment and health from our Mediterranean Diet. In the last chapters we will explore simple and practical steps which can be implemented easily and quickly to make the changes needed to take advantage of this wonderful lifestyle. We will have learned what gives the Mediterranean Diet its "wow factor", and will have illuminated its power through revealing some of its most mysterious secrets.

Summary

The Mediterranean Diet reduces the risk of a wide range of chronic diseases.

The Mediterranean Diet improves mental health, fitness, wellbeing, quality of life and longevity.

The secrets in the diet are not just the ingredients – it is the way they work together in a whole diet.

The health is not just in the macronutrient fats, carbs and proteins – anti-inflammatory and antioxidant compounds you may have never heard of power the diet.

Science is revealing why this ancient diet is the gold standard for our modern world – understanding is the key to unlocking its benefits.

Part One

Understanding the Real Mediterranean Diet

Chapter One

To Begin at the Beginning:
the Story of the Mediterranean Diet

"The Whole Mediterranean, the sculpture, the palm, the gold
beads, the bearded heroes, the wine, the ideas, the ships,
the moonlight, the winged gorgons, the bronze men, the
philosophers – all of it seems to rise in the sour, pungent taste
of these black olives between the teeth. A taste older than
meat, older than wine. A taste as old as cold water."
Lawrence Durrell

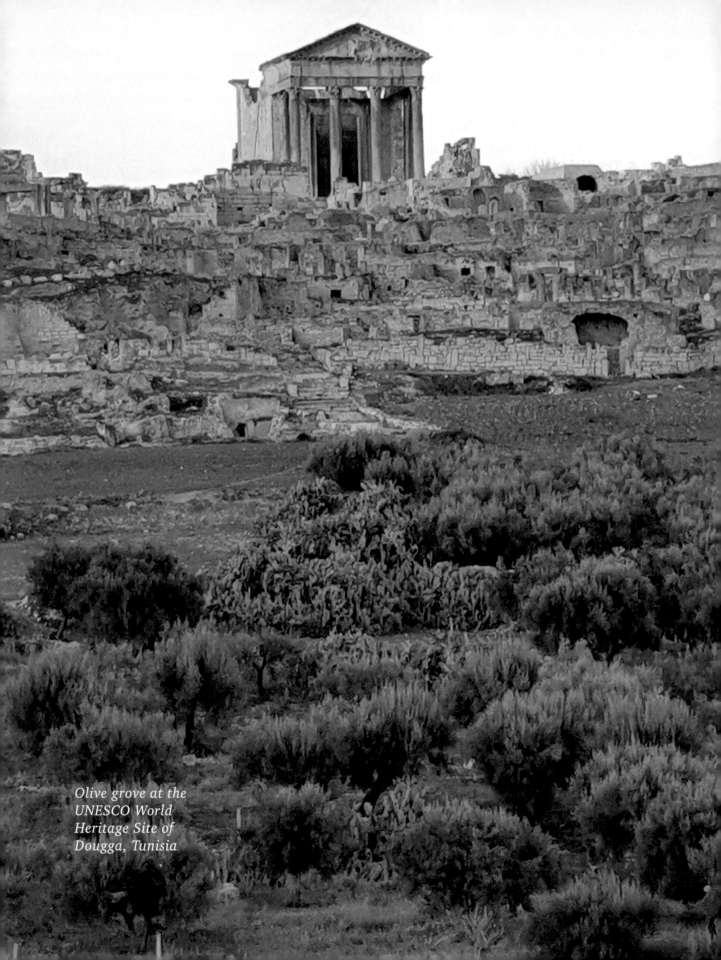

Olive grove at the UNESCO World Heritage Site of Dougga, Tunisia

A Traditional Way of Life

To understand the Mediterranean Diet, we need to know something of its history. The term "Mediterranean Diet" has only been used in the last 70 years, when the pattern of eating in Crete and Southern Italy was recognised by international researchers including Dr Ancel Keys to be associated with a long and healthy life with a much-reduced burden of chronic disease.

Yet the Mediterranean Diet cannot be defined quite so simply. Observing how inhabitants of the region live shows us that the culture of enjoying food is more than can be described by the ingredients alone. The word "diet" is used now to mean a restrictive way of eating to lose weight. This is a departure from its derivation from the Greek word "diaita" which actually means "way of living" and includes strong traditions of regular physical activity, the importance of community, and the time given to eating together. The word "company" ultimately derives from the Latin "com panis" meaning "sharing bread together".

In 2013 UNESCO added this "set of skills, knowledge, rituals, symbols and traditions concerning crops, harvesting, fishing, animal husbandry, conservation, processing, cooking and particularly the sharing and consumption of food" in the Mediterranean Diet to its list of intangible cultural heritage of mankind.

That said, there is no truth to the claim that the benefits of the Mediterranean Diet can only be accessed for those who live in the sunny climes of the region, or that it depends on the genes of those populations. Studies repeatedly show that the benefits from the dietary pattern can be transported very successfully to other parts of the world.

The Lands of the Olive Tree

It would be a mistake to think that there is a single definition of the Mediterranean Diet. Researchers use scoring systems to measure people's adherence to the dietary pattern, giving points to ingredients which characterise the diet. But each region on the shores of the Mediterranean has its own unique version.

For example, the use of herbs and spices, chillies, garlic, wine and different vegetables and methods of cooking vary considerably across countries and the three continents which border the sea. The common feature in the diet throughout the region, and one which defines the edges of lands which describe themselves as Mediterranean, is the cultivation and use of the olive tree.

Evolution and Assimilation

The Mediterranean Diet is not some fad diet or an extreme revolutionary approach to nutrition. In fact, it could be said that it is a way of life which has been refined through evolution over millenia. The origins of this traditional pattern of eating stretch back thousands of years with the transition from hunter-gatherer societies to early settled farming and beyond. That progression has continued through the generations in the cultural melting pot of the Silk and Spice Routes, adding new ingredients from prehistoric times through to the relatively recent introduction of the tomato from the New World and coffee from Africa.

The diet has not only imported valuable flavours and foods which would today be described as the fusion of cuisines – adding spices and fruits such as pomegranate from the east and wholegrains from the west. It has spread beyond the Mediterranean Sea to areas of the New World, near the 40-degree parallel north and south, where the climate can sustain olive trees, wine and other fruits and vegetables of the Mediterranean, bringing the culture to places such as California, South Africa, Australia and South America.

Franciscan monks from Spain planted olive trees in America and nineteenth century doctors such as Penfold and Lindeman from London took vines to Australia to encourage the new settlers to consume alcohol in the more moderate and healthy ways of the Mediterranean. Thomas Jefferson, a Founding Father and third President of the United States of America was a keen farmer, an advocate of healthy eating and had developed a passionate epicurean love for the Mediterranean lifestyle when posted as an envoy of the US Government in France. He tried, unsuccessfully, to plant olive trees on his estates in South Carolina, saying that "of all the gifts of Heaven to man, the olive is next to the most precious, if it be not the most precious."

In Ancient Times

Extra Virgin Olive Oil is inseparably at the heart of the Mediterranean Diet. The first cultivation of the wild olive tree in the Fertile Crescent where farming began was thought to date back to Palaeolithic times, some 7,000 years ago, with organised production of oil from 4,000 BC. However, archaeologists in Israel identified traces of olive oil in containers as old as 6,000 BC. Olive oil had uses not only as a food, but also as fuel for light, soaps and cosmetics.

As civilisations emerged, flourished and declined through the history of the Mediterranean, the importance of nutrition was a constant theme in society. Farming to produce vegetables and grains as well as raising livestock gave a stable supply of food to add to hunting game and the gathering of wild plants.

Foods were identified for their healing qualities including garlic, spices, herbs, wine, and in particular olive oil was observed to have very special properties in ancient texts. From the early beginnings of olive cultivation in the Levant – modern-day Syria, Jordan, Iran and Lebanon, it is thought those prodigious explorers and traders the Phoenicians brought the olive tree and its fruit to their colonies and ports in Southern Italy, North Africa and Spain.

The kings of ancient Babylon created gardens not only for leisure but also to experiment with different edible plants and to explore the health properties of herbs. Doctors were called "Asu" meaning "expert in oil" which may be a reference to the mixing of oil with other ingredients for healing effects.

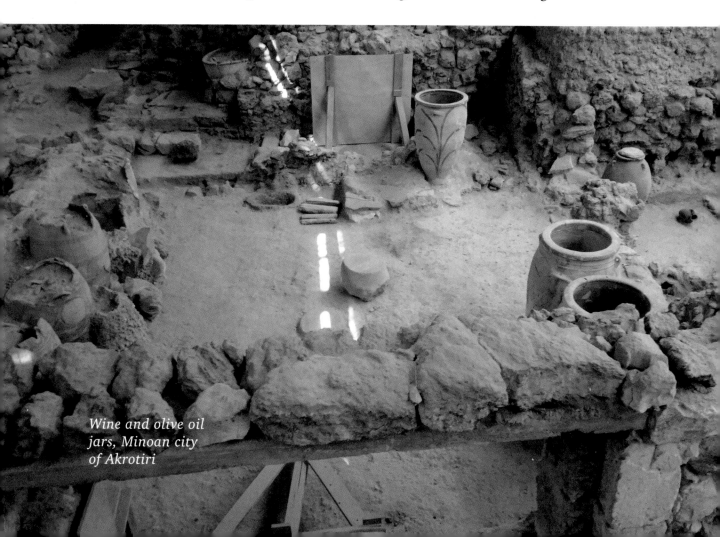

Wine and olive oil jars, Minoan city of Akrotiri

The Great Empires

The Ancient Greeks were not only enthusiasts for the pleasure of eating and drinking, but were also aware of the potential for diet to confer health benefits. Hippocrates wrote "let medicine be thy food and food be thy medicine", recognising that "natural forces within us are the true healers of disease", and olive oil featured in no fewer than sixty of his remedies for various ailments. Dioscórides, a Greek doctor who was a physician to the Roman army recommended the bitter oil of the earliest harvest as a cure for some diseases. It is now known that such oil is highest in anti-inflammatory and antioxidant compounds.

The olive tree was considered sacred in Athenian culture – the symbol of the state and a gift from the goddess Athena in exchange for the citizens' fealty. The writer Herodotus described an incident when the city was burned to the ground by the Persians in 480BC, before Themistocles restored Athenian pride at the battle of Salamis and the inhabitants returned to the Acropolis. It was said that the original and most ancient olive tree of Athens miraculously produced fresh shoots from its charred remains, restoring hope and inspiration to the people.

This should perhaps not surprise us, because olive trees have an extraordinary ability to regenerate, with some of the oldest trees believed to be over 2,000 years old. It is this resilience to environmental challenges which relates directly to the revelations of how the fruit of the tree can have extraordinary powers to protect us and keep us healthy. The Greeks were very familiar with the value of the olive tree. Winners at prestigious games such as those held at Olympia were rewarded with substantial and valuable quantities of olive oil and became the equivalent of modern-day millionaire sports superstars as a consequence.

Some historians have claimed that a significant contributing factor which motivated the Roman invasion of North Africa was control of the fertile plains and in particular the established and highly productive olive groves. Plutarch later praised Caesar's victories on African soil in terms of securing three million litres of oil each year. Writers like Cato and Pliny the Elder produced guides to the production of good quality olive oil and even categorised quality markers which are similar to our modern description of olive oil grades today. Trade in many of the foods we now recognise to be part of the Mediterranean Diet flourished in the time of the Roman empire.

Grains, spices, wine and olive oil were in particular demand to feed the appetites of Rome and to supply the armies at the frontiers of empire. It is still possible today to visit a hill called Monte Testaccio in the capital, an ancient Roman rubbish tip composed almost entirely of fragments of amphorae, the storage vessels for wine and olive oil, many of which contain the stamps of the producers. Quality, provenance and the integrity of products was as important it seems to the Roman authorities as it is to food standards organisations of our modern world.

Gifts from God

Early religious texts make frequent references to foods we associate with the Mediterranean Diet. The Bible and the Koran extolled the virtues of olives, olive oil, grains and bread, bitter herbs and pungent spices, raw honey, grapes, goats' milk, nuts and seeds, fish, vegetables, fruits such as apricots, pomegranates, figs and dates, and passages describe feasts of game and fowl. The ancient olive tree appears in many chapters as a sign of health, peace, hope and fertility.

Recipes for Health from Past to Present

Many ancient texts were familiar to subsequent generations. In particular collections of recipes attributed to Marcus Gaius Apicius were used for centuries after they had been written by this apparently charismatic first celebrity chef of Rome. Similarly, Dioscórides's books describing the medicinal use of more than 600 plants were referred to by physicians well into the middle ages. And so it was that by the 1950s when the American researcher Ancel Keys visited the medieval town of Nicotera, coincidentally built on the ruins of the Greek colony of Medma in Southern Italy, he observed a lifestyle which had been in existence for thousands of years. The Mediterranean Diet was now to be defined in modern terms.

Summary

The roots of the Mediterranean Diet stretch back thousands of years.

The foods and lifestyle of the region have evolved and embraced culinary influences from abroad over generations.

The pattern of life is an intangible part of cultural heritage and tradition.

Olive oil, produced in countries surrounding the Mediterranean and the principle source of fat in the diet has driven economies of empires.

People have long understood the inseparable link between diet and health, food and medicine.

Chapter Two

50 Years of Food Fights

"Do you see over yonder, friend Sancho, thirty or forty hulking giants? I intend to do battle with them and slay them."
Miguel de Cervantes Saavedra, Don Quixote

The Real Mediterranean Diet

A Recipe for Confusion

With continued research during the latter half of the last century showing time and time again the benefits of the Mediterranean Diet, it would seem logical to think that the answer to a healthy lifestyle had been discovered, rooted deep in the people, culture and landscape of the Mediterranean. So perhaps the debate would focus on what makes such a diet uniquely healthy.

And yet when we observe the numbers of diet books available, the contradictory and sensational headlines in newspapers, confused advice from experts, and the highly processed food we are served on our high streets, in supermarkets, schools and hospitals, it would appear that we have learned very little from the evidence available to us.

The Macronutrient Wars

When researchers first described the diet that had been "discovered" in the quiet and unassuming villages in Greece and Italy, the focus soon became fixed on the reported relatively low consumption of saturated fat, considered to be the driver for high blood cholesterol levels which in turn was found to be associated with an increased risk of heart disease through a build-up of blood vessel plaques called arteriosclerosis.

At the same time, there were revolutionary changes happening in food culture in the USA and much of Northern Europe, with the demand for processed, convenience foods rising exponentially. Big business was creating new ways of producing foods to satisfy the desires of consumers and to achieve new "sweet points" of taste which could guarantee repeat sales. Products became increasingly high in sugar, salt and saturated fat and ingredient lists were populated by artificial additives and preservatives.

Instead of looking at the beneficial components of the Mediterranean Diet and how they might work to protect and provide health, the last few decades have seen increasingly polarised arguments about macronutrients in our diet – the fats, carbohydrates and proteins which constitute the majority of our food intake in terms of volume. Food fights – the macronutrient wars – have created the idea of low fat, low carbohydrate, keto and paleo diets, and all manner of variants on those themes with very little focus on the complexity of whole foods and the considerable potential effects on health of nutrients present in smaller quantities. Whilst weight loss for an increasingly overweight population is a laudable goal with undoubted benefits, the focus on body image is a distraction from what a healthy diet should deliver – much broader advantages, protection from chronic diseases and an enjoyable lifestyle which can easily be maintained in the long term. There is compelling evidence to support the role of the Mediterranean Diet for example in the successful long-term prevention, treatment or reversal of diabetes, in addition to being the most effective diet for sustained maintenance of a healthy weight over time. A low carbohydrate diet may also result in weight loss and improve some aspects of diabetes as it reduces refined carbohydrates and calorie intake, but any replacement of poor-quality carbohydrate foods with saturated fat including processed meats, for example, might well increase risk of ill health in the same way that the low-fat mantra of previous times resulted in an increase in harmful processed carbohydrates.

After all, the vegetables, dietary fibre and fruit of the Mediterranean Diet consist of carbohydrates and are associated with significant benefits and deliver many useful micronutrients in their natural forms. There are specific and quite subtle reasons why the combination and interactions of foods in the Mediterranean Diet have been described as the best diet for people with diabetes which will become clear in later chapters. It is a great tribute to the evidence which supports the Mediterranean Diet that whatever nutritional "tribe" commentators belong to, they so often agree that it is a healthy way of eating. Frequently the advocates of low calorie, fasting, low fat or low carbohydrate patterns of eating recommend a Mediterranean style diet as part of the narrative, even if it is not necessarily consistent with the underlying principles of what is being promoted.

Let's Talk About Food

As it happens, the evidence has always supported the rather obvious notion that a good diet depends on the quality and balance of those macronutrients rather than demonising or trying to eradicate one group or another. Food is usually complex and highly variable in its composition which can make these food fights look rather futile and childish. Cheese is an excellent example of how easy it is to get into distracting, reductionist arguments. A question frequently asked is whether cheese is good or bad for health. A processed cheese with emulsifier, added salt, dye and preservative covering a bacon burger is very different from a cave-aged, hand-produced traditional cheese eaten with figs or grapes. There are subgroups of saturated fats present in cheese and these vary in their effect on cholesterol. For example, the saturated fats of the fermented milk of goats and sheep are considered to be less of a concern when it comes to their effect on cholesterol levels than those found in milk from cows. Cheese is an important source of calcium and vitamin D for many. A healthy and diverse population of gut bacteria which we now know to be essential for health may be supported by regular, moderate consumption of cheese. So, in the final analysis, the answer to whether cheese is good or bad for health may depend on the type, quantity and quality of cheese and the circumstances in which it is eaten.

When arguments are based on false or oversimplistic assumptions it is no wonder that there is fertile ground for further confusion. There is money to be made with health claims on foods and supplements or in controversial new books and on social media.

Unfortunately, this is made even more muddled by official systems such as "traffic light" nutritional labelling which fail to make distinctions between different subclasses of macronutrients and have no ambition to describe micronutrients and bioactive compounds which may be beneficial.

There is something of Don Quixote in the story of recent debates around nutrition. The deluded knight of Cervantes's original tale perceived an enemy in windmills, which occurred to him as malign giants to be defeated. Separating macronutrients such as fats or carbohydrates from the context of the whole food matrix and the complex relationship between ingredients, making no distinction between different types, and declaring them to be the enemy sets the stage for a similar battle in an unreal landscape with predictable farcical results.

This can only be countered by consistently citing the evidence and explaining the reasons for the incomparable power of the Mediterranean Diet – a whole diet which begins and ends with food in the context of a healthy lifestyle.

Debates about the effects of macronutrients such as saturated fat and carbohydrates swirl around us. There are continuing arguments about diets for weight loss and contention on the subject of the importance of cholesterol. Meanwhile there has been a much more significant advance in our understanding of human health and illness which relates to how chronic diseases begin and are propagated.

Inflammation – The Root Cause of Chronic Disease?

Inflammation appears to play a crucial role in chronic disease. Our dietary choices have a profound influence on stoking or quenching the fires of inflammation in our bodies. It is the micronutrients and bioactive compounds in foods which may have the most important role to play through anti-inflammatory and antioxidant effects.

Summary

Most of us know what a good diet looks like, but confusion still surrounds us.

Conversations about diet get stuck with macronutrients – we should be talking food.

Conversations about diet get stuck with what we shouldn't be eating.

It is more relevant to talk about the nutrition of how whole foods come together in a diet.

Chronic diseases may be driven by chronic inflammation.

Chapter Three

Inflammation – We Know What Makes Us Sick

"No disease that can be treated by diet should be treated by any other means."
Moses ben Maimon

A Revolutionary New Theory of Disease

It is now recognised that many chronic diseases are inseparably linked with long term destructive inflammation. Coronary heart disease, stroke, many chronic respiratory conditions, diabetes, dementia, obesity and some types of cancer have now been categorised as diseases of chronic inflammation. Three out of five deaths in the world today are due to these illnesses and the World Health Organisation describes them as the greatest threat to human health. It is not surprising therefore that if we can find a lifestyle which supresses the fire of chronic inflammation then it has the potential to dramatically and positively change the health of billions of people.

We can take heart disease as an example of how thinking has changed. Previously it was believed that if we ate too much saturated fat, cholesterol plaques would form in the blood vessels of the heart and this "furring" would eventually block the crucial blood supply to the heart. We now understand that it is in fact inflammation of these cholesterol deposits which is more important. As the injurious plaques threaten to damage arterial walls, inflammation occurs as a natural response and if unchecked and uncontrolled this can lead to the formation of a blood clot called an embolus which in turn can have devastating effects of interrupting blood supply to the heart.

These effects are not confined to the heart. The same processes can affect blood vessels which supply other parts of the body and can lead to strokes, common forms of dementia and kidney disease for example.

Chronic inflammation is also believed to be linked to the development of up to a third of cancers, where it can disrupt the normal functioning of DNA – our genetic blueprint which programmes the behaviour of cells, resulting in uncontrolled growth of tumours.

Some conditions such as arthritis which are linked to chronic inflammation may be driven by genetic factors and a misdirected immune system damageing the body's own cells. Increased risks of heart disease are observed in individuals with arthritis due to this inflammatory state, even though symptoms are primarily experienced in joints. Some medications with an anti-inflammatory effect like aspirin have been used to prevent heart attacks, strokes or some types of cancers.

Paradoxically, drugs which where promoted for a particular reason are now being found to work because of their effect on inflammation. Statins, for example, may exert more powerful effects as "stablisers" of the inflammatory processes associated with high cholesterol rather than simply in reducing its levels.

Diet and Inflammation

Diet is an important factor which can influence chronic inflammation. We now know that some foods have extraordinarily healthy anti-inflammatory effects in our bodies, whereas some are capable of inciting inflammation. Saturated fat, refined sugars and meat can be pro-inflammatory in their effect. High and spiking circulating blood sugar levels, diabetes and obesity are pro-inflammatory states. Insulin, the hormone responsible for processing sugar, becomes less effective in these circumstances resulting in a vicious pro-inflammatory circle called insulin resistance.

Alcohol in moderation can have an anti-inflammatory effect, but in excess is pro-inflammatory. Calorie restriction and fasting create an environment of lowered inflammation whereas the complex and very necessary chemistry which occurs to metabolise the foreign material necessary for life we call food increases inflammatory responses. The omega 3 fats in oily fish and some plants including nuts can be converted into substances called resolvins which as the name suggests resolve some aspects of inflammation. Plant rich diets which include vegetables, fruits, wholegrains, nuts and seeds contain very many powerful anti-inflammatory elements and can even moderate the results of foods which are pro-inflammatory.

Researchers have defined a "Dietary Inflammatory Index" – the "DII" – to measure these effects and rank dietary patterns. A diet which has a low Dietary Inflammatory Index correlates with much reduced rates of chronic diseases. Studies are showing particularly significant effects of such diets on reducing the risk of cancers. A lower DII diet has also been demonstrated to improve mood. The Mediterranean Diet has a very low DII and is therefore amongst the healthiest of ways of eating when it comes to inflammation.

To understand how the Mediterranean Diet promotes healing and reduces chronic inflammation as the best example of an anti-inflammatory diet, it is first important to understand the role of inflammation in health and the bioactive components of foods which can protect from disruptive chronic inflammatory processes.

Understanding Inflammation – The Good and the Bad

Inflammation is, on the one hand, a natural and protective reaction. In response to acute injury or invading bacteria or viruses, our bodies have evolved mechanisms of defence. Acute inflammation involves the production of powerful chemicals which attack and destroy these pathogens. Victory over a potential breach of our healthy state depends on the mobilisation of our immune system, assigned to seek and eliminate the threat. This often results in temporary damage of our own cells as well as those of our enemies, with swelling and heat contributing to the successful rout of the incursion. As the body returns to normal, reconstruction and repair occurs with a return to a state of health. We exist in a delicate balance between protective inflammation designed to destroy infections and our internal balance of healing once the danger has passed.

Chronic inflammation however can have very negative effects, with collateral destruction without the chance to heal. Sometimes it is not entirely clear what leads to chronic and uncontrolled inflammation. There are some obvious triggers such as pollutants and external toxins including smoking for example which set off inflammatory responses. Our genes and our capacity to control our own immune response can also play a part. Obesity and some foods are intriguingly also associated with increased levels of chronic inflammation, often low grade but potentially lethal over time. The word itself derives from the phrase "to set on fire" and like fire, inflammation can wreak havoc if not controlled. But as we will see, there are also ways in which those fires can be suppressed or extinguished.

Measuring Inflammation

There are methods to measure inflammation through chemical markers in the blood. These indicators of inflammation have names such as C- Reactive Protein, TNF-alpha and IL-6. These are sometimes used to monitor the activity of inflammation. In a clinical setting they are often raised significantly above normal levels in acute infections or chronic inflammatory diseases such as arthritis. Although we do not need to understand the details of these indices of inflammation, we will see their relevance in appreciating the effects of the Mediterranean Diet in "The Sofrito Story" later in this chapter.

Powerful Chemistry – Theories of Inflammation and Oxidation

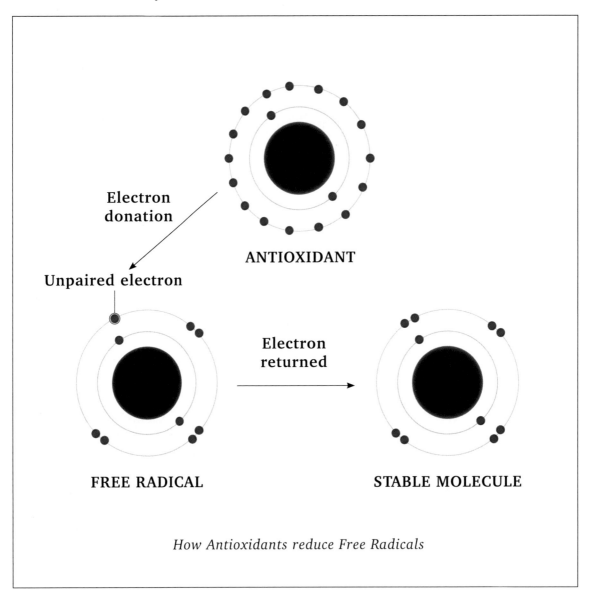

How Antioxidants reduce Free Radicals

The chemistry of inflammation is complex, but it is really important to understand in order to appreciate its game changing effects, and the basics can be explained fairly simply.

An important element in natural processes, including inflammation, is oxygen. Oxygen is a highly reactive atom. It is fundamental to life. We breathe in its most common paired atom form known as O_2 to use it in cells to create the energy we need to live. We can see the power of oxygen all around us in its ability to rust metals, or to change the exposed flesh of an apple in minutes. These reactions are called oxidation and the substances with which it reacts are described as being oxidised.

Oxygen is also a powerful ally to call on for its potentially destructive properties in fighting off infections, and its reactive effect can be a potent force to eliminate pathogens. When oxygen appears in its particularly powerful "reactive oxygen species" or "ROS" form it is chemically charged, with unpaired electrons and in need of scavenging electrons from other molecules to become stable. It is a "free radical" and is not satisfied until it has searched out and replaced its missing electron, stealing from other molecules, which in turn breaks and disrupts them, resulting in a chain reaction of destruction. This "oxidative burst" can be invaluable when unleashed by immune cells on invading bacteria or viruses and we can create these free radicals to defend ourselves. This reactive power, however, needs to be harnessed and regulated for healing to occur.

In very small and controlled ways free radicals can also be produced and used in other normal cell functions. The domino effect of the unbalanced charge of a free radical seeking to pair its electrons from other molecules can be used for internal cell chemical messageing systems, the controlled passing of electrons being comparable to the passing of a baton in a relay race. Another good analogy is to compare it with the way that we can control potentially destructive nuclear reactions with internal and external oversight designed to safely create electricity.

Similarly we have evolved chemical systems which might involve a gentle ripple effect of limited use of free radicals in cells or create a brief and focused inflammatory tsunami to flood an encroaching infection in a defensive emergency.

However, it is the ability to regain balance and healing which restores good health, and puts an end to the acute inflammatory effect when it is no longer needed. The targeted killing of cancer cells through the production of free radicals by radiotherapy is a way this power can be used in medical techniques in a similar way to the body responding with oxidation as part of the acute inflammatory response. But without management and constraint free radicals can be destructive. Free radical producing radiation can on the one hand kill cancer cells, but if exposure is uncontrolled it can actually be the cause of cancers.

Oxidising free radicals are not only part of the process of protective acute inflammation and well controlled internal systems. They are also formed as unwanted by-products of normal cell processes and metabolism, or from negative environmental factors such as smoking, pollution or radiation. If their levels cannot be controlled they can be harmful and potentially damage our cells and organs. This is referred to as a state of "oxidative stress".

Our ability to manage the effects of oxidation are finely tuned, with rebalancing "redox" systems working to maintain a healthy state. However, when the fires of chronic inflammation are burning, we may need the support of natural anti-inflammatory and antioxidant agents, many of which can be available in a healthy diet. These plant-based compounds are sometimes called "free radical reducers". Our bodies have adapted so that unwanted and potentially harmful free radicals can be mopped up and neutralised by vitamin E for example and stored safely in fat tissues before being transported out of our bodies by water soluble antioxidants such as vitamin C. Other very important protective compounds we get from our diets are called polyphenols. In an experiment, children can be shown at home, lemon juice and extra virgin olive oil each preserve an apple from the browning effects of oxidation. This is through the antioxidant effects of Vitamin C in the lemon juice, vitamin E in olive oil and the numerous antioxidant polyphenols in both.

Polyphenols are not what most people in nutrition circles talk about. They are not like the familiar carbohydrates, proteins and fats, which make up the largest proportion of our food intake. But size does not necessarily count for much when it comes to powerful effects on health. So important are the antioxidant and anti-inflammatory effects which may protect us from chronic diseases including heart disease and cancers that we will learn more about polyphenols in a chapter entirely dedicated to the most important things you eat you have probably never heard of.

Meanwhile let us take this theoretical chemistry of oxidation and inflammation and put it in a real-world environment and consider how these effects can be seen in daily life.

The Sofrito Story – polyphenols at work

Sofrito is a wonderful combination of extra virgin olive oil, tomatoes, onion and garlic rich in antioxidant and anti-inflammatory compounds.

It is a tradition in Spain to have a breakfast comprised of this pungent, tasty mix of ingredients on warm toast, washed down with strong coffee. It is also used as a base for many sauces. It has been used in some of the scoring questionnaires as a measure of how closely people adhere to the principles of the Mediterranean Diet. The consumption of sofrito is associated with improved parameters of heart disease risk and increased sensitivity to the hormone insulin, which in turn has a protective effect against obesity and type 2 diabetes. The Italians have their own version sometimes made with peppers or celery, called soffritto.

Researchers have identified numerous individual polyphenol compounds in the ingredients of sofrito. There have been thirty-six discovered in extra virgin olive oil alone. Sofrito contains active ingredients with exotic names such as naringenin, ferulic acid, and quercetin as well as tyrosol and hydroxytyrosol and other polyphenols from extra virgin olive oil.

A rather simple but cleverly designed study has recently shown that if individuals are fed a diet low in polyphenols for a few days and then consume a single meal with sofrito, they show a dramatic increase in polyphenols which can be measured in their urine, but most importantly they have significantly lowered blood levels of the markers of inflammation C-Reactive Protein, TNF-alpha and IL-6. This shows the potential for powerful effects of dietary polyphenols controlling and lowering levels of inflammation. Dousing the flames which burn.

And of course, it also demonstrates how immediate this effect can be which means that each day we might be able to reduce the levels of chronic inflammation in our bodies. It might also explain why time after time research has shown that adopting a Mediterranean Diet can have benefits within weeks, and that there is no age at which it is too late to see those advantages. It should make us think of how today's meals are affecting our bodies today rather than believing that our state of health is set in stone or solely and irreversibly determined by a misspent youth.

A Sofrito Side Story

As it happens sofrito has also been the subject of research into the interrelations between the ingredients, which has wider implications and shows how important it is to consider the health effects of nutrients in whole foods (the so-called food matrix) rather than just the macronutrients. Even this is not enough – we need to understand how the constituents of foods affect each other and how our body responds to these interactions when foods come together in meals.

Cooking sofrito in extra virgin olive oil increases the availability for absorption of many of the micronutrient compounds in all the ingredients. Sometimes this is simply because those important anti-inflammatory and antioxidant chemicals are fat soluble and so dissolve into the cooking juices with the olive oil, and sometimes there are more mysterious factors at work.

For some compounds which might only be available in very small quantities otherwise, mixing with extra virgin olive oil appears to greatly increase their ability to be absorbed. The transfer and mixing of polyphenols between the tomatoes, garlic, onion and extra virgin olive oil when cooked together in sofrito is a dance of chemistry which can be seen in other meals where extra virgin olive oil is a key ingredient. The accessibility for absorption of these polyphenols in extra virgin olive oil as part of a unique food and meal matrix may be one of the secrets of the power of the entire Mediterranean Diet.

Summary

Inflammation is a natural way to destroy infections but chronic inflammation can be damaging to our own body.

Levels of chronic inflammation can be measured.

Oxygen free radicals are powerful chemicals disrupting others in what are called oxidation reactions as part of inflammation.

Nutrients in our diet can have pro-inflammatory or anti-inflammatory effects.

What we eat today influences chronic inflammation today.

Chapter Four

Polyphenols – Nature's Answer to
Chronic Inflammation?

"Natural forces within us are the true healers of disease."
Hippocrates

Polyphenols – 21st Century Nutrition

Let's face it, if you went to a bar for a drink or a restaurant for a coffee, you would be unlikely to hear much conversation about polyphenols. Yet If you were to look at the scientific papers published on the subject you could find extraordinary discoveries and suggestions that these plant-based compounds have powerful effects which can influence health and disease. Most books on diet and lifestyle do not mention polyphenols. Even in scientific debate they remain more a side show rather than the star attraction, although that is changing as their importance is recognised.

Polyphenols contribute positively to lowering a diet's inflammatory index, as well as playing a major part in a food's ability to neutralise free radicals. This is measured as the ORAC score – the Oxygen Radical Absorbance Capacity, although because this is a laboratory measurement, we cannot necessarily assume that we can apply these scores in real life. That said, recently the Total Antioxidant Capacity of a diet – the TAC score, has been shown to be predictive of a longer, healthier life with comparable accuracy to other more established diet quality measures.

The Known Knowns and Known Unknowns

Scientists are a little cautious about pronouncing these bioactive compounds a panacea for health, and that is to be respected. There is certainly scope for more intensive research and there is much yet to be discovered. Acknowledging areas where more investigation is needed is an integral part of the journey of developing scientific knowledge, and any nutritional recommendation which asserts absolute certainty or makes exaggerated claims should be treated with great caution.

There are legitimate questions about how available these compounds are to the body and how they are altered by our gut bacteria, and whether it is those products of bacterial processing which have an effect. There are differences between what can be observed "in vitro", meaning in laboratory test conditions compared with our ability to prove their effects "in vivo" which is to see changes in our physiology in real life.

Given the difficulties with clearly seeing antioxidant effects in the body, there are different theories about how exactly they might work. Some evidence suggests that their antioxidant effects may occur mainly in the gut while other research provides insight into the possibility that even with a low measurable antioxidant effect once digested and absorbed, the antioxidant effect on a cellular level might be quite powerful after all. Polyphenols and their metabolites might be more absorbed when combined with fellow polyphenols, work synergistically, and even form networks through which they might recharge each other, enhancing their capacity. Some theories suggest that they have more of an effect on genes or that they modify other aspects of chronic inflammation rather than directly through antioxidant effects. Polyphenols may work in all these ways with a combination of direct and indirect antioxidant activity, activation and regulation of other aspects of inflammation processes or through influencing the way our genetic programming is expressed.

The way we handle bioactive compounds such as polyphenols may also be quite personal and at least to some extent dependent on genetics as well as our gut microbiome – the term used to describe the microbes living in our gastrointestinal tract, the pattern and diversity of which has a powerful effect on health and can change over time. There is cutting edge research into such genetic variability and debates about the importance of "precision nutrition" to understand what this means for us as individuals.

There is a lot we still have to learn about the many thousands of polyphenols thus far identified. Rather than be frustrated that it is not possible to describe their effects in simplistic ways, the many mechanisms by which they might work should be a reason to celebrate the role they can play in health. The known unknowns should not deter us from taking the knowledge available to us and using what we know to improve our health.

It is also important to resist the temptation to try to short circuit millennia of evolution by imagining that separating chemicals with antioxidant properties and combining them in a pill will have the same beneficial effects as those contained within the food matrix. Supplements simply do not cut it. In general, despite a thriving market in antioxidant pills and capsules, it is hard to find any evidence to support their use. Often the contents of a supplement are poorly absorbed because they are fat soluble and the original food would have been eaten with a meal with fat and then refined by the bacteria in our guts. In some experiments the addition of concentrated antioxidants appeared to have the opposite of the intended effect and cause harm, perhaps through the dose and formulation overwhelming and disrupting the body's own redox systems, resulting in a damageing prooxidant rather than antioxidant effect. Polyphenols can also, in excessively high supplement doses, reduce the absorption of other important vitamins and minerals. Yet despite the remaining mysteries, there is clear evidence that plant polyphenols from foods in our diet can have powerful positive effects for health. This rises above the "antioxidant hype" and emphasises the importance of consuming polyphenols as part of a balanced Mediterranean Diet.

Polyphenols – A Family of Fascinating Compounds

Polyphenols are present in many forms in plants and have antioxidant effects. There are lots of subgroups of these chemicals with names such as flavonoids, phenolic acids, stilbenes and lignans. Some may be familiar to us such as tannins which are antioxidant polyphenols found in tea, or curcumin present in turmeric. Some plants produce quite specific polyphenols and their names often reflect where they are most commonly found. For example, limonene is a polyphenol in citrus fruits, rosemarinic acid is found in herbs including rosemary, and piperine in pepper.

Polyphenols are particularly abundant in fruits and vegetables, extra virgin olive oil, olives, wholegrains and legumes, teas, coffee, dark chocolate, honey, wine, herbs, spices and nuts. It is probably no coincidence that this quite accurately describes the Mediterranean Diet. It is estimated by some researchers that the Mediterranean Diet has three times the total polyphenol quantity when compared with a standard western diet although other studies have found similar levels of total polyphenols especially in populations who drink a lot of tea and coffee. Perhaps more important than the total level is the greater variety and complexity of the polyphenols in the Mediterranean Diet, including those unique to extra virgin olive oil, how they combine together in meals and their abundance in seasonal foods . It may be that the diversity of polyphenols contributes significantly to the health benefits and the anti-inflammatory effects of the foods associated with the Mediterranean Diet. Is this the clear blue water separating diets, and putting the Mediterranean Diet so far ahead?

Antioxidant Healing – How Polyphenols May Work for Us

Despite the challenges of understanding their absorption and of clearly seeing polyphenols at work in the body, there is convincing evidence that diets like the Mediterranean Diet that are rich in polyphenols protect from chronic inflammation and chronic diseases. The predominant theory of how this occurs is through the "biochemical scavenger theory" - a process by which the polyphenols or their metabolites once absorbed mop up damageing free radicals and incorporate them into stable molecules.

Free radicals are atoms or molecules which are unstable. In short, they lack electrons. Electrons generally like to be in pairs and a free radical has one or more unpaired electron. We can look upon that free radical as aggressively

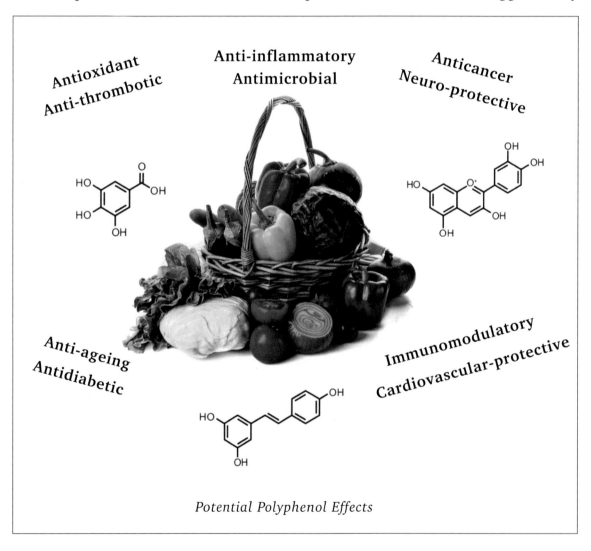

Potential Polyphenol Effects

seeking to stabilise itself by stealing an electron from another molecule, perhaps injuring and destabilising the structure of that molecule and in turn setting off a chain reaction, inflicting further destruction on others. Although this can be useful to the human body, it can also be very damageing, where it is uncontrolled, resulting in "oxidative stress". DNA within cells and fats which protect the integrity of cell walls are particularly vulnerable to oxidation, the latter producing more unstable molecules called lipid peroxides which continue the cycle of damage.

Oxidative stress is not only a feature of chronic inflammation which is associated with chronic diseases like heart disease and cancers but it is thought also to contribute to damage in nerve tissue associated with Alzheimer's Disease, be part of the toxic effects of excess glucose in the body in people with diabetes and also align with factors which predispose to weight gain. Some researchers believe polyphenols are therefore important in preventing illnesses which we might not normally immediately associate with chronic inflammation such as dementia, diabetes and obesity.

Polyphenols have rather complex formulae in the textbooks of chemistry. They are hexagonal rings made up of carbon, hydrogen and oxygen atoms. But for the purposes of this book, all we need know is that phenol rings are generous donors of electrons. They can withstand giving up electrons to free radicals, quenching their thirst, stabilising them and potentially limiting their damage.

Polyphenols have been shown to have antioxidant and anti-inflammatory effects with anti-cancer, anti-hypertensive (protection from high blood pressure), anti-thrombotic (prevention from blood clotting), antidyslipidaemic (protection from high cholesterol) and antimicrobial effects (protection from infection). They are protective to the nervous system and the heart. Studies involving foods rich in polyphenols such as Extra Virgin Olive Oil, fruits including berries, spices, red wine and cocoa have demonstrated and replicated many of these therapeutic effects.

We Lead Stressful Lives

Life involves chemistry, reactions and energy. This inevitably produces the oxidising free radical by-products which can cause the damage and disruption to cells known as oxidative stress.

It has been suggested that the state of sleep is the time when there is least oxidative stress. It has even been suggested that one of the purposes of sleep is to provide the opportunity for the body to rebalance that oxidative stress. Perhaps the beneficial effects of a siesta might be ascribed to the chemical "rebooting" to a state of lowered stress.

After eating, when the body is presented with food, there is a great deal of chemistry required to process, metabolise and store the new compounds as useable material for the vast numbers of functions needed to sustain life. In particular the rise in sugar levels and the absorption of saturated fat following a meal is known to cause oxidative stress. As we eat frequently during the day unless we are fasting, our body is said to be in a state of post prandial oxidative stress for much of the time. The body has its own internal systems to reduce oxidative stress but there is increasing evidence that the polyphenols present in food play a vital role in mitigating and reducing the metabolic prooxidant effects of eating. The inclusion of polyphenol rich vegetables and other ingredients in a meal with fruit as a desert have been shown to be important in reducing markers of post prandial oxidative stress and inflammatory effects.

If the production of free radicals is a consequence of chemical reactions in the body then vigorous exercise might be expected to yield a state of extreme oxidative stress. Yet we know that exercise results in very great advantages to health. It is believed that this is because exercise produces the most efficient and effective response the body can muster to rebalance the stress with targeted and powerful internal redox systems. Following the effort of exercise there is a clear net gain, with the rapid restoration of a state of increased insulin sensitivity, reduced oxidative stress and inflammation. It is perhaps not surprising that there are evolutionary mechanisms in place to resolve the challenge of exercise but not yet the negative effects of a relatively recently adopted modern unhealthy, prooxidant diet.

Polyphenols in Nature – Nothing is Coincidence

Polyphenols are present in many plants available for us in our diet. The antioxidant effects which we can harness are of course there to serve a purpose to the plant itself. The reactive nature of oxygen and oxygen free radicals poses a risk to plants. We can often see the effects of oxidation on the flesh of a fruits and vegetables which have been exposed to the environment just for a few minutes. This process is even more rapid where there is light and heat. So, the plant defends itself by producing polyphenols, often most abundantly in the outer covering most exposed to the elements. The skin and external layers of fruits, vegetables, nuts and the husks of grains are especially rich in polyphenols. It is interesting to observe that this is particularly the case with nuts which contain polyunsaturated fats which are most susceptible to oxidation. The bark, roots and leaves of plants are often the original source of polyphenol rich spices and herbs.

At the same time as protecting the plant from oxidation, polyphenols often combine their antioxidant power with antimicrobial properties, conferring protection against attack from harmful bacteria or viruses. Often polyphenols give the colour to fruits. As a fruit develops and matures to a state where it is ready to be consumed in order that its seed is distributed, changes to colour may occur, signalling to an animal or bird that the fruit is ripe and ready for eating. Polyphenols are concentrated in the purple of blueberries, the redness of an apple and the green hues of an olive.

Sometimes plants produce polyphenols which have a particularly bitter or pungent taste to animals in order to protect the plant from being eaten. Where a tree is in symbiotic relationship with a creature which might eat its fruit and helpfully distribute the undigested seed for propagation, when the right degree of maturity is reached there may be an increase in the sugars or fats which make it good for eating, which often coincides with a reduction in the protective and bitter polyphenols. If the fruit is not eaten at this stage it may soon decay with the effects of the environment. Some plants, for example chilli and olive trees have even managed to create polyphenols in fruits with properties which make them less palatable to some species, whilst birds which are the preferred carriers of their seeds are impervious to the pungent or bitter tastes. The range of seed distribution may be increased in this way with less competition for scarce resources with the parent plant.

Nature, in polyphenols, can be seen at her most ingenious. Plants exist in a dynamic relationship with their environment and this dictates the purpose and effects of polyphenols.

Tasting for Polyphenols

Polyphenols often have bitter, spicy or pungent tastes. Taste enjoyment is a matter of individual preference but also can be developed over time. These attributes can add flavour and interest to food and we can learn to love them and enjoy the potential health benefits.

For example, high levels of capsaicin in chilli peppers provide antioxidant capacity and cause a burning sensation, which for many people enhances their experience of food.

Rocket (arugula) leaves in a salad contain many polyphenols which are called flavanols and provide an astringent sensation, bitter or "peppery" taste.

The antioxidant polyphenols in herbs and spices often have their own unique combinations of flavours.

Dark chocolate which contains high levels of cocoa such as at concentrations of seventy percent or more is bitter but better, containing higher levels of polyphenols than lower concentrated chocolates.

Espresso coffee for the same reason is bitter, but has a higher ORAC score than other milder tasting brews.

Olive oil can be bland and rather uninteresting in flavour when it is refined or simply rather low in natural antioxidants. Bitterness and pungency along with fruitiness are considered positive attributes for a good extra virgin olive oil, and the taste directly reflects the polyphenol levels and therefore the health benefits of the oil.

Production and Preparation for Polyphenols

Since polyphenols are produced for protection against oxidation and disease which is more likely in extremes of light and heat, plants have learned to respond to a more demanding environment by ratcheting up the levels of polyphenol antioxidants when needed. In other words, "stressed" plants may produce fruits with higher levels of polyphenols. Varieties of species which have evolved in regions where conditions are harsher may also have adapted by raising their production of polyphenols. This has quite extraordinary implications. It means that the way in which we farm our food can have very significant effects on polyphenol levels. For example, there is evidence to suggest that grapes which grow in difficult environments with little irrigation, at altitudes with higher UV light exposure and with extremes of temperature, produce more of the peppery procyanidin polyphenols in wine which may have a beneficial effect on the heart.

Aged wine tends to have reduced levels of its original procyanidins, although if it is stored in oak barrels it is possible to identify polyphenols from the oak which suffuse into the wine and may play a role in taste and health. The plant which contributes most to the Mediterranean Diet has been the subject of much research into the way production changes chemistry, and we will explore this in more detail in the chapter dedicated to extra virgin olive oil – a very significant source of polyphenols in the diet.

Manufacturers of foods are not permitted to make health claims on the basis of polyphenols, not because they are not good for us, but due to remaining uncertainty about variation in levels, the possibility of differences in the way they are metabolised by our differing colonies of gut microbes and the challenge of demonstrating the effects of individual polyphenols in particular foods. That said, researchers are leading the way with extra virgin olive oil, where one particular group of polyphenols, when present above a set minimum amount, has successfully been granted the rarefied status of a health claim by the European regulatory authorities.

Polyphenols – Nothing Lasts Forever

Polyphenols are able to counteract the chemistry of oxygen, especially in its most reactive form as free radicals or Reactive Oxygen Species. As we exist in an oxygen rich environment capable of creating the energy we need to exist and light the fires of metabolism, there is constant pressure on polyphenols to absorb the oxidative stress of the world around.

This means that polyphenols will inevitably over time give up their antioxidant capacity if exposed to oxygen, light and heat. There is only so much generous polyphenol donation of electrons that can be sustained. Eventually their protective antioxidant properties will diminish and plant material will begin to degrade and deteriorate into rancidity. Unless preserved, the potential power of polyphenols as anti-inflammatory and antioxidant bioactive nutrients will be lost.

Summary

Polyphenols serve the plant to reduce the damage from reactive oxygen in the environment, protect from microbial attack and unwanted attention from herbivores.

Plant polyphenols act as antioxidant and anti-inflammatory compounds in human health and reduce oxidative stress.

Polyphenols often give fruits and vegetables their vibrant colours and taste – hints of bitterness and spice.

Plants respond to environmental challenge by producing more protective polyphenols.

The Mediterranean Diet is uniquely rich in dietary polyphenols.

Chapter Five

The Mediterranean Diet
How and Why it Works

"Everything you see I owe to spaghetti."
Sophia Loren

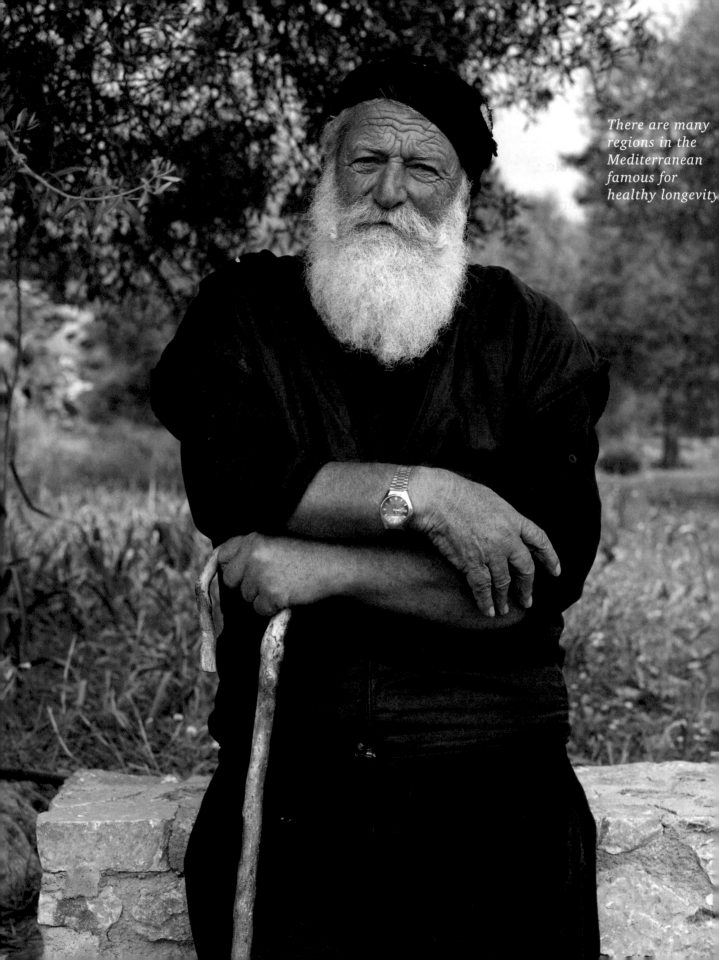

There are many regions in the Mediterranean famous for healthy longevity

The Miracle of the Mediterranean Diet

As we learn the way in which the healthy, polyphenol rich, anti-inflammatory Mediterranean Diet works to protect from chronic diseases, we can build a more complete picture of the foods which make up the diet. The evidence shows that the methods of preparation, cooking, and the combination of ingredients create many of the added benefits.

Plentiful multi-coloured vegetables either raw in salads or cooked with extra virgin olive oil are the foundation of the diet. Wholegrains and legumes are staples, with herbs and spices punching taste and health above their weight. Fruit is generally enjoyed after a meal and a handful of unsalted, raw, skin-on nuts may be commonly consumed each day. Olives are a frequent snack or are mixed with other foods in meals. Extra virgin olive oil, in significant quantities, is used in every aspect of the cuisine. Fish, eaten once or twice a week is cooked in extra virgin olive oil and free roaming poultry or game is also part of the diet. Unprocessed honey is generally used as a sweetener. Water is the drink of choice, although wine is often taken with a meal and herbal teas through the day. There is moderate consumption of eggs with yoghurt and cheeses, generally from the milk of sheep or goats also included. Desserts and red meat appear much less frequently on the menu.

The Mediterranean Diet Adherence Scores used by scientists to measure the effect of the diet when compared with other patterns of eating use many of these features to positively or negatively score levels of alignment with the Mediterranean pattern of eating.

The Mediterranean Diet has an incredibly broad beneficial effect. Research over decades has revealed consistently positive results. Studies have involved observing and comparing different patterns of eating and some have looked at populations that have been randomly selected to follow the Mediterranean Diet to compare the difference with another diet. We have a good idea of how much reduction in relative risk of various chronic diseases there is when we have a Mediterranean Diet. It is important to understand the idea of relative risk because a large percentage figure reduction is much more meaningful for a disease which has a common prevalence or background risk. A sixty percent reduction in not very much, is not very much.

A thirty percent reduction in something very common is more significant. There is a difference between absolute and relative risk. Of course, there is a difference between association and causation, the latter not necessarily being proved by the former. However, if results repeatedly show alignments such as we see with the Mediterranean Diet and reduced chronic disease and we have a plausible theory to explain the link, then it is quite literally a matter of life and potentially preventable early death that we understand and can make the changes to our lifestyle.

Nutritional science is not easy to conduct accurately. Robust research depends on successfully excluding so called confounding factors – aspects which might be associated with outcomes and co-exist in the studies, perhaps becoming confused with the subject of the study. Higher numbers of participants in studies yields greater confidence in the results. Many of the publications on the Mediterranean Diet have included meta-analysis which involves number crunching several studies to draw even more reliable conclusions and can bring the number of participants effectively studied to as many as half a million.

Studies large and small, short term and long term including those with names such as PREDIMED, EPIC and SUN have all shown reduced risks of many chronic illnesses where people follow the diet. These even include results where changes are made late in life. Reduction by as much as a third in relative risk of many diseases has been shown including heart disease, heart attacks, strokes, many different types of cancers, dementia including Alzheimer's disease as well as obesity and diabetes. Kidney disease, blood pressure and some eye conditions are also significantly improved with the adoption of the Mediterranean Diet. The effects of inflammatory conditions such as arthritis, inflammatory bowel disease like ulcerative colitis and asthma are all mitigated.

Some studies have included death as an outcome over a measured period of time, and for the length of the research, data has shown a substantial reduction in mortality.

Mental health, cognitive function, well-being and quality of life parameters are also dramatically improved with the Mediterranean Diet.

One of the largest randomised controlled trials, PREDIMED, was forced to stop before the planned completion date because the benefits of the Mediterranean Diet were clearly so strong that it was deemed unethical to continue to have a group taking a non-Mediterranean Diet. They were informed that there was already sufficiently compelling evidence that they should at once convert to the healthier Mediterranean Diet. The study had by that stage shown a thirty percent reduced risk of cardiac events, strokes and overall mortality, and a sixty percent reduction in rates of breast cancer. The data continues to be analysed and is revealing further positive news on the incidence of cancers, obesity, diabetes and dementia.

Publications sometimes draw fascinating and unexpected conclusions. It seems that if you live in Manhattan, are eighty years old and consume a Mediterranean Diet you are more likely to have a larger brain. And if you are from the Greek island of Ikaria in your sixties, consuming the Mediterranean Diet with olive oil, you are twice as likely to have a good sex life, it appears through having better blood vessel health where it matters.

There are numerous studies to show that the advantages are just as powerful in populations who do not live in the Mediterranean region. It is not dependent on genetic stock or fine weather though both may play a part in good health. Data from Northern Europe, Australasia and the USA demonstrates the gains are just as valuable in other parts of the World. There is a particularly rich seam of evidence coming from an ongoing study of New York firefighters who are learning about, and benefitting from the Mediterranean Diet.

Modelling using existing data has shown that a combination of lifestyle factors which include adherence to the Mediterranean Diet has the potential to add between 8 and 15 years of life.

It is no wonder that the Mediterranean Diet since it was first observed has amassed a vast database of research and is now recognised for its role in significantly improving health and longevity.

Getting the Basics Right

The Mediterranean Diet represents all that we know to be good in nutrition. It is unprocessed, healthy and sustainable.

Although it is much more useful to focus on whole foods rather than macronutrients, so much debate revolves around macronutrients that it is worth briefly considering this subject before moving on to more interesting aspects of the Mediterranean Diet. It is not a low-fat diet. It is not a low-carbohydrate diet. The key is the "quality" of those macronutrients.

There are four groups of fats most relevant to health; transfats, saturated, monounsaturated and polyunsaturated fats. Transfats are harmful and associated with heart disease and have been present in many processed products and food from fried food outlets. They exist in negligible quantities in the Mediterranean Diet. When it comes to saturated fat the story is more complex because there are different subtypes of saturated fats, some associated with raising cholesterol levels and others with little or no effect. The saturated fat in the Mediterranean Diet tends to be from the fermented products of sheep and goats in the form of cheese and yoghurt containing saturated subgroups which are not considered to be unhealthy. It is believed that the fats derived from animal meat are more likely to have a negative effect than those of dairy products. There are generous amounts of monounsaturated fats in the Mediterranean Diet, mainly from olive oil which has a beneficial effect on cholesterol levels. The majority of the fat in olive oil is in monounsaturated form and is called oleic acid or sometimes referred to as omega 9 fat. Awareness of the health properties and stability of oleic acid has led producers of sunflower oil and peanut growers to create high oleic acid variants of these plants so that their foods may be promoted for their high oleic content. Polyunsaturated fats in the form of omega 3 and omega 6 fatty acids can be healthy, but only if consumed in the right proportion because they compete with each other in some aspects of their effects. Excesses of omega 6 fats can result in a pro-inflammatory effect. Like saturated fats, polyunsaturated fats are therefore something of a mixed bag.

Western diets tend to have a ratio of sixteen to one of omega 6 to omega 3 polyunsaturated fats, largely because of the consumption of vegetable oils high in omega 6 fats and a lower intake of omega 3 rich foods such as oily fish, nuts, seeds and green leafy vegetables. The Mediterranean Diet has an ideal ratio closer to four to one not only because fish, nuts and greens are staples in many parts of the region, but also because olive oil is used as the main source of fat for cooking rather than omega 6 heavy vegetable oils.

Carbohydrates and sugars are usually low glycaemic index (GI) in the Mediterranean Diet. This is good for health, avoiding undesirable spikes in blood glucose. The glycaemic index of a food mainly comprised of carbohydrate is a measure of how quickly the sugars are absorbed and released into the blood stream. The term glycaemic load (GL) is used to describe the sugar release of a combination of foods. The body handles dietary sugar absorption by mobilising the hormone insulin to ensure that it is appropriately taken out of circulation to be stored for energy use. Habitual intake of high GI carbohydrates results, to put it simply, in a "tiring" of the insulin response (known as insulin resistance or decreased insulin sensitivity) which can result in obesity, type 2 diabetes and the proinflammatory effects of raised circulating blood sugar levels. The low GI carbohydrate nature of the Mediterranean Diet allows for the benefits of high vegetable and wholegrain intake with sugars locked in complex, "slow release" carbohydrates which are known to be rich in beneficial nutrients including vitamins, minerals, polyphenols and fibre whilst avoiding weight gain and diabetes. Food combinations common in the Mediterranean Diet are also important in affecting the glycaemic load of a meal, emphasising again that it is over simplistic just to consider macronutrients alone without understanding the context of foods and meals. Similarly, when considering a diet high in simple sugars or vegetable oils it is not only necessary to consider its effect on a person's weight, but more importantly the direct results on levels of inflammation.

Proteins in the Mediterranean Diet are more plant-based than in our red meat rich western lifestyle. In particular legumes such as beans, chickpeas, lentils and peas are frequently included in dishes from the region adding important micronutrients as well. Traditional lifestyles could not afford the regular consumption of red meat as a protein source, reserving it for feast days or other celebrations. Fish, poultry and dairy products are eaten in moderate amounts and also provide good quality protein.

Digging Deeper – Polyphenols and Other Bioactive Nutrients

Although the food fights continue, the basic principles of good nutrition are reasonably well established as long as we talk of whole, natural food.

In some respects, this makes the Mediterranean Diet simple to understand on a superficial level. It contains the right combination and quality of macronutrients and is low in refined sugars, preservatives and additives. It is unprocessed and based on "real food". It is high in fruit and vegetables. It is low in red meat, excess intake of which has been associated with an increased risk of cancer. If we look deeper than the macronutrients it is a diet rich in important vitamins, minerals and fibre, all of which are important for human health. The combination of foods does not need long ingredient lists with unrecognisable chemicals. In this diet there are no powder supplements, no shakes or "bullet proof coffees". A tomato is a tomato. An onion is an onion.

However, the key to unlocking the real power of the diet is in understanding and applying the principles which decrease chronic inflammation.

Polyphenols and other so-called bioactive nutrients from plants, collectively called phytonutrients can have important effects to decrease chronic inflammation and to potentially reduce oxidative stress and damage. For the sake of completion, some bioactive substances with antioxidant effects fall outside the classification of polyphenols. Glucosinolates present in garlic and broccoli, carotenoids in carrots and other yellow or orange foods and Vitamin E all have antioxidant effects, as well as the more familiar Vitamin C. Polyphenols, however, are consumed in much larger quantities – typically ten times the amount of Vitamin C and one hundred times that of Vitamin E and carotenoids put together.

Bioactive compounds are present especially in the rainbow of colourful foods, may vary depending on how the food is produced, and often appear in those ingredients we might add to increase flavour, such as herbs and spices. It would be possible for a person to believe mistakenly that they were achieving the benefits of the Mediterranean Diet as simplistically described in some articles if they were eating a few more vegetables with poor quality olive oil, occasional fruit and reducing meat consumption. It is, however, the more subtle effects of the wide variety of foods, their quality, taste, the effects of combining ingredients, the way of cooking and their micronutrient content which really turbocharges the effects of the Mediterranean Diet. The catalyst for this is frequently the combination of foods with the ever-present extra virgin olive oil. This is where the alchemy of the Mediterranean Diet occurs and this is considered in more detail in the next chapter.

Those Old Men and Women of the Mediterranean – How Do They Look So Great?

We can all recognise the archetypal image of the elderly inhabitants of a small hillside Mediterranean village, sitting and gossiping on the bench. They lean on their walking sticks and gaze at their sixty-year-old sons and daughters hard at work in the olive grove and listen to the bells of the churches and the goats. There is an intangible relationship between the land, the people and the foods that sustain them. This relationship seems intuitive and is "the natural way of things".

The number of people who enjoy a longer and healthier life in the region is much higher than in other parts of the world. To some degree this may reflect the protective factors of an environment where there is importance attached to the community and family. Regular exercise and an outdoor life with lower levels of stress and pollution may also have a part to play. Diet is certainly absolutely central.

The Mediterranean Diet has been shown to contribute significantly to healthy ageing. This is of course an inevitable consequence of the lower levels of chronic diseases and the protection from heart disease, stroke and cancers. Studying centenarians, that is those people who have reached the age of one hundred, reveals that they are more likely to have a Mediterranean style diet and also have measurably lower levels of inflammatory markers detected in their blood. Researchers have described the fourfold increase in number of centenarians in a mountainous region in western Sicily and attributed their health to an active lifestyle and low glycaemic Mediterranean Diet with fruit, vegetables and extra virgin olive oil rich in polyphenols.

There is also evidence from studies in the Mediterranean region and other parts of the world including the USA that the diet improves brain function in the elderly, even if it is adopted late in life. This includes reduced rates of Alzheimer's Disease where the formation of damaged tangles of brain tissue may be prevented by elements in the diet.

And what of ageing itself? Scientists have described how, as our cells divide and we age, the protein caps which sit at the ends of strands of our DNA genetic blueprint become shorter. These caps called telomeres – markers of ageing, are longer and more preserved in individuals following the Mediterranean Diet.

Oxidative stress is a major factor in the processes of ageing in all organs of the body including the largest and most visible – the skin. Whether it is the effects of smoking, ultraviolet light exposure or diet, signs of skin ageing are most obvious in a state where oxidative stress is unchecked.

The Mediterranean Diet for a Healthy Weight

The traditional Mediterranean Diet of previous generations is consistent with a healthy weight. Unfortunately, many people of the region have adopted the processed and "fast food" culture of the West, and obesity and diabetes are a growing problem.

Research shows that adopting a traditional Mediterranean Diet results in a steady and consistent move towards an ideal weight. The beneficial effects gradually overtake the weight loss of other diets such as low carbohydrate, keto, Atkins and low fat when studied in comparable circumstances. The typical pattern of a loss of effect over time seen with other diets is not observed with the Mediterranean Diet, not least because the diet is so enjoyable and satisfying that people remain faithful to it rather than giving up.

There are a number of reasons why it is consistent with a healthy weight.

Although it is relatively high in fat, the presence of extra virgin olive oil encourages a feeling of fullness. Foods in the diet are low GI and extra virgin olive oil itself when combined with carbohydrates reduces sugar spikes by slowing absorption and increasing insulin sensitivity resulting in less risk of weight gain. Some polyphenols have been shown to have anti-obesity effects.

Extra virgin olive oil, whilst a fat with higher calories per gram than proteins or carbohydrates, is not associated with weight gain despite a substantial amount consumed in the diet. It has been confirmed that it does not result in the laying down of abdominal fat.

Calorie counting, though it is used in studies comparing diets for weight loss, is not as useful in regulating food consumption everyday as considering modest portion sizes and the quality of meals.

Eating food for enjoyment and in company tends to make meals last longer. It has been observed that this style of eating results in the chemical messages of fullness having time to reach our brains.

A Healthy Mind

The Mediterranean Diet is associated with better mental health. Studies have revealed that you are less likely to suffer with depression the higher your Mediterranean Diet adherence score.

Although it is hard to precisely define wellbeing, people are more likely to report positive social functioning and feelings of vitality with good physical and emotional health when they more closely follow the diet.

What Will You Feed Your Gut Bacteria on Today?

In the last ten years we have seen much more interest in those trillions of bacteria which naturally inhabit our gut. There are books devoted entirely to the subject of the gut microbiome. In short, a diverse population of good bacteria in our gastrointestinal tract has an important effect on the nutrients absorbed and the refining of the foods we eat. This has widespread effects including our risk of disease, inflammation and on our mental health. A highly processed diet results

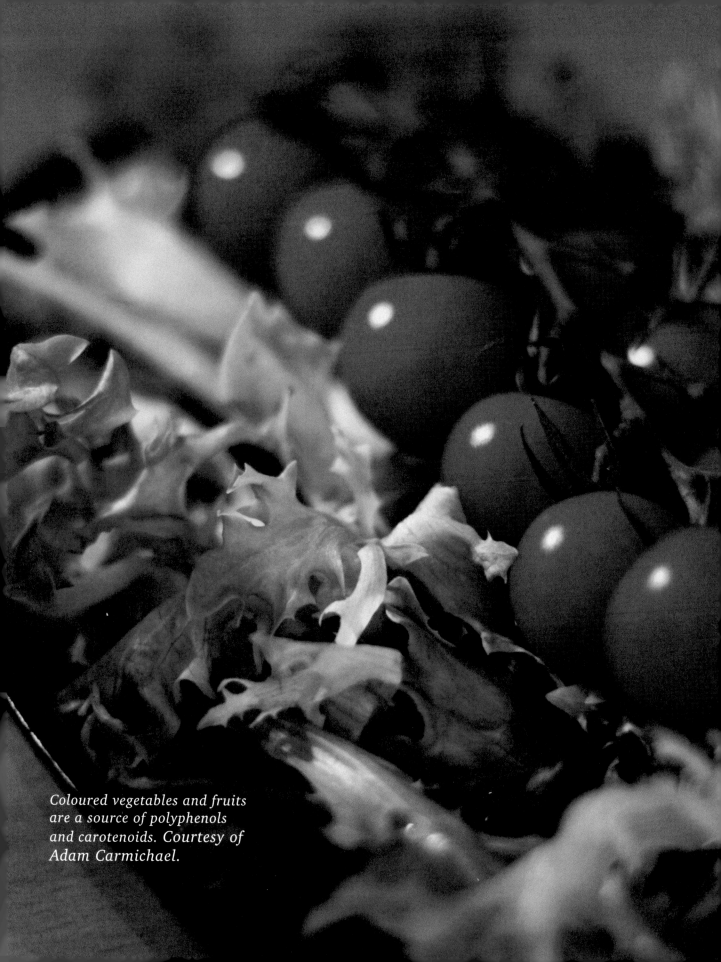

Coloured vegetables and fruits are a source of polyphenols and carotenoids. Courtesy of Adam Carmichael.

in less varied gut microbial colonies with a lower proportion of the most helpful bacteria with which we have a symbiotic and mutually beneficial relationship.

Vegetables, pulses, fruit and nuts have all been proven to be associated with a healthy gut microbiome. Fermented foods, sourdough breads and fibre are also favourable. Gut bacteria seem to be particularly partial to the polyphenols in extra virgin olive oil. Regular consumption promotes a diverse microbiome with species of bacteria which have been shown to influence many aspects of health including our mental wellbeing.

The so-called gut-brain axis describes the relatively new discovery that our gut bacteria are important in the production of chemicals which positively affect our mood. A diet rich in polyphenols, a significant proportion of which are available in our large intestine to promote a healthy microbiome can positively improve our mood. This may explain the reason why the Mediterranean Diet is associated with significantly better mental health.

The Mediterranean Diet is a perfect diet to maintain our friendly gut bacteria. We might consider ourselves farmers of our gut microbiome. We can nurture them well through the food choices we make.

Body Communication Systems – More Dots Joining Up

Having thought that the organs in our body have distinct functions which they get on with performing in isolation, scientists are beginning to realise that there are multiple ways in which the different systems are in contact with each other. Just as we know that the mind and the gut are in constant chemical conversation, there is also evidence that a hormone called osteocalcin which is produced in response to exercise helps not only strengthen bone and muscle and regulates glucose metabolism but also seems to be related to preserving mental agility in older age. Osteocalcin has been found to be significantly more abundant and active in Mediterranean Diets with extra virgin olive oil. This is perhaps another way in which the diet exerts its anti-ageing effects, though more research is needed to understand exactly how.

Power over Genes

Another exciting frontier of science is the study of epigenetics. It was once thought that the genetic code in our DNA dictated our life course in an inflexible way rather like the Fates of Ancient Greek mythology predetermining our journey.

Epigenetics is the study of the interactions which can affect our genetic blueprint. It turns out that the "expression" of genes, in other words how much they influence our lives, can be altered by environmental factors including diet. The effect of nutrients on gene expression is called nutrigenomics. Since our genes are quite individual there is interest in understanding whether people with specific genetic profiles are more or less affected by this interrelationship. It is clear that there are differences in the way we respond to particular foods although this is surpassed by the incontrovertible evidence of the benefits of the Mediterranean Diet as a healthy way of eating.

A Mediterranean Diet can increase the expression of good genes which have a positive effect on health and can even "switch off" genes which, for example may be associated with increased inflammation or risk of heart disease. Extra virgin olive oil polyphenols have even been cited as possible inhibitors of genes linked with cancer cell replication and growth as well as genes involved in the damage of blood vessels.

Extra Virgin Olive Oil – At the Heart of the Mediterranean Diet

Many populations of the Mediterranean eat as much as three times the quantity of vegetables compared with those living in other countries. They also consume ten times the quantity per capita of extra virgin olive oil. As one lead Greek researcher said; "it is not perhaps that we in Greece like vegetables more than people living elsewhere, it is that we are able to make exquisite meals through combining them with copious amounts of extra virgin olive oil"

If there are two key ingredients of the Mediterranean Diet, they are probably vegetables and extra virgin olive oil.

Summary

The evidence for the benefits of the Mediterranean Diet is well established and incontrovertible.

The Mediterranean Diet gets the basics of macronutrient balance and quality right.

The Mediterranean Diet does more than protect from diseases, it promotes healthy ageing and mental health.

The Mediterranean Diet is excellent for gut health and the microbiome.

The Mediterranean Diet promotes healthy expression of our genes.

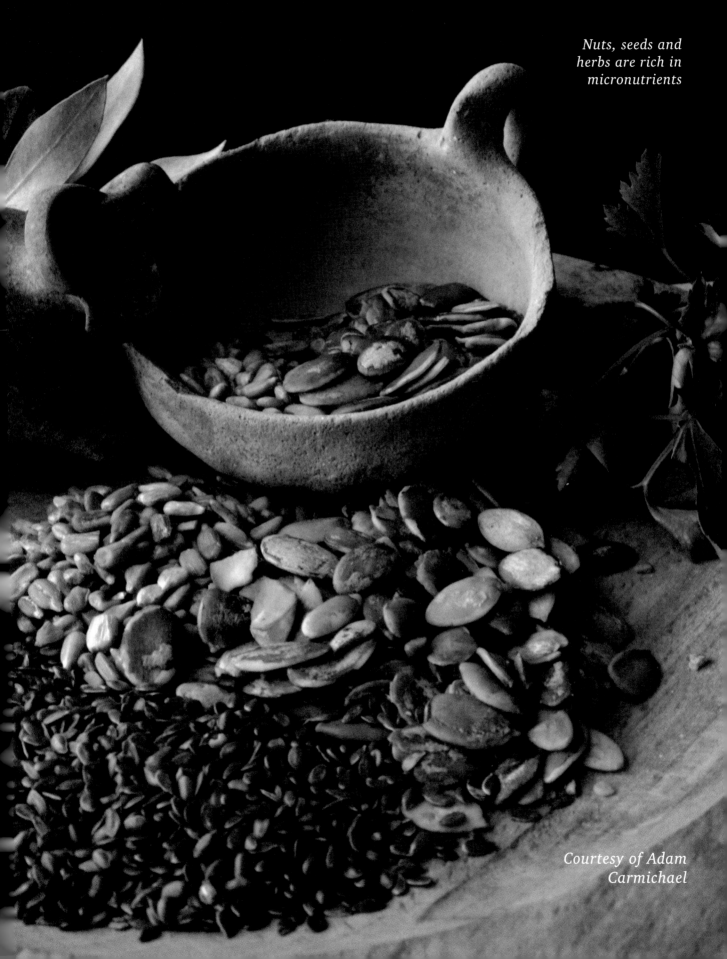

Nuts, seeds and herbs are rich in micronutrients

Courtesy of Adam Carmichael

Chapter Six

Extra Virgin Olive Oil
Central to the Mediterranean Diet

"The riper the berry the more greasy and less pleasant the flavour of the oil. The best time for gathering olives, striking a balance between quality and quantity, is when the berries begin to turn dark."
Pliny the Elder

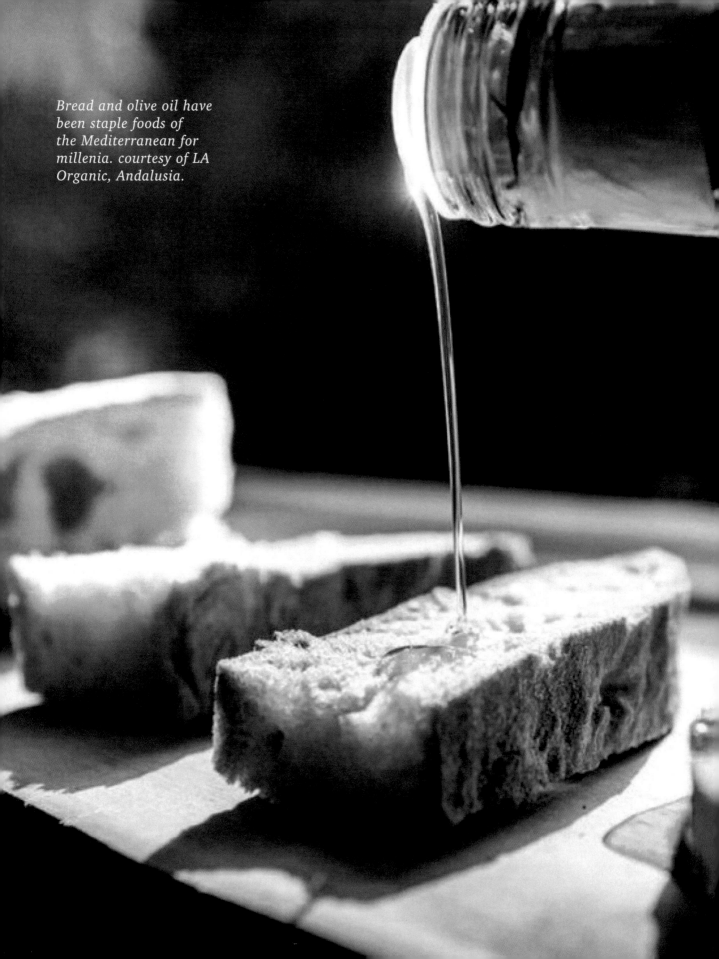

Bread and olive oil have been staple foods of the Mediterranean for millenia. courtesy of LA Organic, Andalusia.

Ubiquitous Extra Virgin Olive Oil

The traditional diet of Crete was one which was described as a typical regional variant of the Mediterranean Diet. In this diet it was said that forty percent of total calories came from fat and that the majority of that fat was from olive oil.

This is a very substantial proportion of any diet, and no single ingredient anywhere in the world has such primacy and dominance in a diet. It is ubiquitous in the Mediterranean, and olive groves often stretch as far as the eye can see. It is used for food preparation, marinating and mixing, as the only cooking oil, and for dressing and adding flavour and texture to finished meals. It is used in the kitchen and for "anointing" dishes. It can be found in large cans in the larder and in bottles on the tables of every typical Mediterranean household.

Extra Virgin Olive Oil in Mediterranean Culture

It is difficult to describe what olive trees and olive oil mean to the inhabitants of the region. They are so deeply rooted in the culture of the Mediterranean. Festivals and religious celebrations are dedicated to the olive harvest. Growers are passionate about their trees and the quality of their extra virgin olive oil. The olive tree has shaped the history of our world and continues to change the landscape. The olive tree advances on its journey to grace the lands of the New World and the Southern Hemisphere as more people begin to understand the gifts of health it bestows on humankind. It is possible to see goats climbing the lower branches of a tree in Morocco and kangaroos grazing on olive leaves in Southern Australia.

Extra Virgin Olive Oil in the Mediterranean Diet – Considerable, Independent and Measurable Effects

It is self-evident that extra virgin olive oil is central to the Mediterranean Diet, but this is also backed up by the science. When researchers look at the effects of the diet and find the extraordinary benefits, they usually use scoring systems which, for example, may weight vegetables, fruits and other staples with positive scores from zero to three. The regular use of olive oil in many recognised scoring systems counts for as much as the consumption of vegetables. This is often defined as the inclusion of olive oil in every meal. Where evidence associates the reduced risk of chronic diseases with a high Mediterranean Diet score it is always the case that olive oil will be contributing significantly to the score. It is impossible to take olive oil out of the science of the Mediterranean Diet. There is certainly no justification for any suggestion that an alternative cooking fat could be used to achieve the effects of the Mediterranean Diet.

There is increasing evidence that shows extra virgin olive alone has positive measurable effects on health. This is quite a feat given that it is often hard to separate fact from fiction in a world where there are so many challenges to producing good quality nutritional science. To be able to identify so many benefits in a single ingredient is quite remarkable and unique.

There is a 40% relative reduction in risk of strokes associated with regular consumption of olive oil. A Mediterranean Diet with high polyphenol extra virgin olive oil showed on ultrasound the visible regression and healing of damaged areas in carotid arteries with improved blood flow. Two tablespoons of olive oil each day correlates with a 44% reduction in rates of heart disease. Regular consumption of olive oil reduces the risk of diabetes by between 50 and 80% depending on the population studied. Extra virgin olive oil has been shown to have effects on blood cholesterol, the oxidation of cholesterol, the health of blood vessel walls and their elasticity, blood clotting, anti-cancer properties and a protective role in some autoimmune diseases including inflammatory bowel disease and arthritis.

How Much Extra Virgin Olive Oil?

It is interesting to look at the typical quantity of extra virgin olive oil measured in research which records the benefits of the Mediterranean Diet and of extra virgin olive oil alone. This would suggest how much we should consume each day.

Studies on average cite the use of between 30mls and 50mls of extra virgin olive oil per day. There does not seem to be a maximum level that should be consumed as part of a well-balanced diet.

To put this into perspective this consumption is typical of the populations of Italy and Spain. The Greeks have traditionally consumed as much as 70mls per day. A conservative estimate of what we might aim for in the lower part of the range to have an adequate Mediterranean Diet equates to approximately twelve litres per person per year. This is still only half of the intake of a citizen of Greece. Currently the average consumption in most non-Mediterranean countries including Northern Europe and the USA is less than one litre per year per person. Yet this is what we should consume each month to match the Mediterranean Diet adherence scores which align with much better health. A key to understanding and achieving the real Mediterranean Diet is learning the pleasures of incorporating considerable amounts of delicious extra virgin olive oil into the meals of every day.

Changing the Paradigm – A Daily Staple

If we wish to follow the Mediterranean Diet it can be seen that we need to on average increase our extra virgin olive oil consumption by a factor of ten. It is useful to look at the practicalities of this.

As people learn to enjoy using extra virgin olive oil every day to roast, fry, prepare food, marinate, baste, drizzle and add for flavour and texture as they do in the Mediterranean, the ways in which we buy oil inevitably changes.

When we shop, we tend to associate certain foods with a particular frequency of purchase. Fresh vegetables are usually bought each week and one or more bottles of wine might also be considered to last a few days at most, but a bottle of extra virgin olive oil is often regarded as a monthly purchase. A large bottle of extra virgin olive oil would easily be consumed in an average household each week for the application of the Mediterranean Diet.

Alternatively, larger quantities of extra virgin olive oil can now easily be bought to last several weeks or a month or two. Three and five litre cans or boxed oil can be sourced at very reasonable prices and decanted into other receptacles for everyday use.

Extra Virgin Olive Oil – For the Polyphenols

Extra virgin olive oil is essentially a freshly squeezed fruit juice. It consists predominantly of cholesterol friendly monounsaturated fats. It is also a good source of Vitamin E. However, it is the polyphenols which are most important for their extraordinarily positive effects on human health.

Extra virgin olive oils are in general rich in polyphenols, though the actual amounts can vary. It is important to note that the lesser grades of olive oil have lower levels or are devoid of polyphenols. By definition oils which do not meet the chemical or sensory standards of extra virgin olive oil are lacking in polyphenols. There are a number of ways to define extra virginity but the simplest is by a measure of acidity. The fats in the form of fatty acids in the oil are bound together in groups of three called triglycerides. If there has been oxidation then these break up and the fatty acids become free, increasing the measured acidity of the oil. Polyphenols will have inevitably sacrificed themselves in the fight against oxidation. Extra virgin olive oils are required to have acidity levels below 0.8% which reflects the preservation of polyphenols. They have lower levels of free fatty acids and are less oxidised. To produce extra virgin olive oil great care has to be taken to reduce oxidation, thereby preserving the stable triglycerides and polyphenols. Virgin oil is oil from the press which does not meet the standards of extra virginity, having higher levels of acidity though still below 2%.

A bottle which is labelled "olive oil", with no mention of virginity, consists of oil from the mill of such low grade that it requires refining through heat to make a flavourless and odourless fat fit for consumption. Such oil is likely to be low in polyphenols in the first place and the operation of refinement results in further inevitable loss. There is a small amount of extra virgin olive oil added back to give some flavour before sale. Levels of polyphenols in refined olive oil are therefore very low. Pomace oil is an even lower grade of oil extracted through industrial methods from the olive flesh and stones after previous pressing.

A virgin or extra virgin oil is uncontaminated and unsullied by processing or interference, its integrity and purity remaining intact – hence the name. This can be demonstrated not only in its taste through experienced tasters, but also in chemical analysis, usually identifying chemicals including polyphenols with a laboratory spectrophotometer which identifies the presence of compounds through the absorption of UV light.

At the time of writing there are thirty-six polyphenols so far identified in extra virgin olive oil with names such as oleuropein, oleocanthal and hydroxytyrosol.

We are at the beginning of a fascinating journey of discovering the possible activity of each of these components. There are challenges in understanding how these compounds are changed by our gut microbes and absorbed. Scientists can measure the amounts in foods and often find polyphenols in appreciable amounts in our urine, but it is often difficult to see them at work in our bodies.

In laboratory experiments oleuropein has been shown to have powerful antioxidant activity against cancer cells. When fed to animals bred with a predisposition to dementia it markedly reduces the formation of tangled nerve plaques similar to those seen in Alzheimer's disease as well as preserving their ability to perform cognitive tasks.

Oleocanthal has anti-inflammatory effects similar to ibuprofen and is antioxidative, antimicrobial, inhibiting of cancer cells replication, and demonstrates neuroprotective activities in laboratory studies. It has been reported to suppress melanoma, breast, liver, and colon cancer cell growth. It also appears to have the ability to help clear damageing protein seen to be laid down in nerve tissues in Alzheimer's disease and may have a protective effect against Parkinson's disease.

Work is going on to establish exactly how these effects might work in humans but it certainly appears that the levels of polyphenols are crucial. Researchers are beginning to compare low polyphenol and high polyphenol extra virgin olive oils and demonstrating that the higher the polyphenol level the greater the beneficial effects. In one such study individuals with early Alzheimer's disease were given an extra virgin olive oil specifically selected for its high polyphenols and showed much improved mental functioning compared with those consuming a diet with lower polyphenol olive oil.

We know that meals such as sofrito will decrease markers of inflammation and a similar experiment has shown that consuming extra virgin olive oil high in polyphenols achieves the same effect.

Hydroxytyrosol is one of a number of polyphenols unique to extra virgin olive oil and olives which has powerful antioxidant effects which can be seen affecting factors which are directly associated with heart disease. We now know that heart disease is driven largely by inflammation and the accompanying oxidation of LDL cholesterol plaques in our blood vessel walls. Levels of antioxidant hydroxytyrosol or compounds related to it in good quality extra virgin oils can reduce the damageing effects of this process and by implication protect the heart. The evidence is so convincing in human studies that the European regulators of food health claims allow producers of extra virgin olive oil with a certain minimum level of hydroxytyrosol to describe this "reduction in oxidative stress" on LDL cholesterol on their labelling, though few consumers are currently likely to comprehend the implications unless they have read and understood such ideas.

We are witnessing polyphenols in extra virgin olive oil becoming recognised for the part they play in the effects of the Mediterranean Diet.

Factors Determining Polyphenol Levels

Challenging environmental conditions demand more protection from oxidation. Stress experienced by the olive tree will maximise polyphenol production, and levels will diminish when the olive is ripe and ready for dispersal.

There are over 700 varieties of olive and some naturally produce more polyphenols than others. Varieties such as Picual and Koroneiki for example tend to produce more polyphenols.

Olives harvested earlier will have higher levels. As it ripens an olive turns from green to purple and oil levels will increase as polyphenols reduce. The earlier harvest oils will be richer in polyphenols although the amount of oil will be less.

If a grove is heavily irrigated and water is plentiful, the trees are less stressed and produce lower levels of polyphenols. Though the farmer will benefit from a greater yield, the quality of the oil will be lower from the perspective of health and also by virtue of a blander taste. A hot and dry climate will, in contrast, produce oils with higher levels of polyphenols.

Organic cultivation may increase the stress on a tree, thereby inducing higher levels of polyphenols, because there is less reliance on artificial methods of combatting microbial attack.

Factors in the soil can also have an influence on polyphenol levels – the terroir and other features of local geography.

The general consensus is that olive trees are capable of growing at altitudes of 1200 meters above sea level for commercial purposes though this is dependent on local factors and olive tree cultivation has been attempted at altitudes much higher than this in places such as Nepal. There is increased ultraviolet light at higher altitude which increases oxidative stress and results in the need for the olive tree to increase polyphenol levels to protect its fruit.

Once harvested, oxidation by heat or light with the presence of oxygen in the environment will result in the depletion of polyphenols as they disperse the effects of reactive oxygen. A similar effect occurs if the olive is damaged or invaded by microbes.

This means that the processes of harvesting, collection, transportation, milling, storage, bottling and preparation for collection by the consumer need

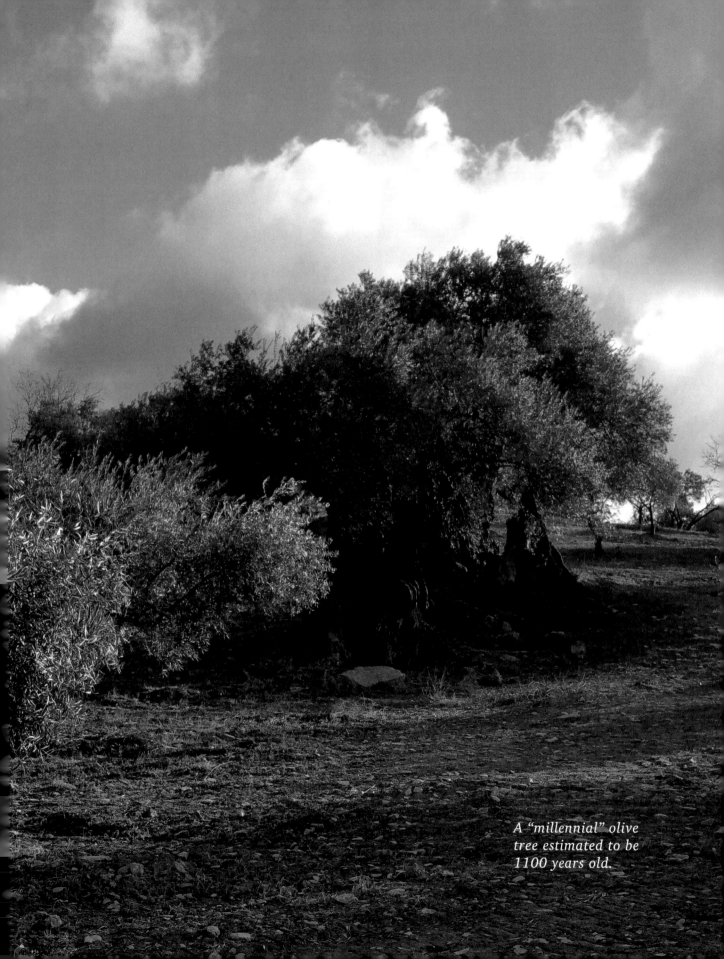

A "millennial" olive tree estimated to be 1100 years old.

to be careful, efficient and cognisant of the effect of the factors which can diminish the quality of the oil and be detrimental to the polyphenol levels and ultimately result in rancidity.

Tasting the Difference – The Sensory Revelation

Good quality extra virgin olive oils are renowned for their fruity aroma and flavours. Tasting oils has become an art for some, and there are sommeliers of extra virgin olive oils just as there are for wine. The smell of freshly cut grass, herbaceous notes, almonds, green bananas and ripe tomatoes are just some of the descriptions used by connoisseurs to assess the harmony and complexity of smell and flavour. Degrees of bitterness and pungency are also considered positive attributes for an oil, with varying intensities from a mild or sweet oil to the most robust, peppery and spicy oil.

The bitterness and pungency of an extra virgin olive oil relate directly to the polyphenol levels. We know that polyphenols in plants frequently possess bitter characteristics and once we have learned to enjoy and value these tastes and sensations, we can choose oils which we know are very healthy. For example, oleuropein has a bitter taste and oleocanthal gives pungency to an oil and is the chemical associated with the cough that may be caused by some oils through a mild and transient irritation of the throat.

Nature has provided us with the ability to recognise an oil that is good for us. We can try different oils at home and soon understand how to identify healthy oils.

Of course, a sweet and gentle, less bitter oil may be a good choice for some tastes or with milder, more delicate dishes whilst stronger, peppery oils are reserved for other meals. The point is that we know how to recognise the polyphenols and to make choices accordingly. Olive farmers can, within the constraints of the varieties and the geography of their groves, make decisions about their agricultural techniques, time of harvest, care of processing and varietal blending to create different quality and tasting oils. There may be an early harvest, higher polyphenol, lower yielding oil which might be chosen as a premium product early in the season, to be followed by the pressing of a second quality oil later in the month.

Cooking for Health with Extra Virgin Olive Oil

Extra virgin olive oil is the best choice to use in cooking. We sometimes hear it said that it should not be used in cooking because of its "smoke point". This is simply not true. Given that it is the only oil used for cooking in the traditional Mediterranean Diet, if it were anything but beneficial to cook with it, the diet simply would not work. It cannot make sense that a fundamental part of the Mediterranean Diet is anything other than advantageous.

The "smoke point" is the temperature at which an oil burns or produces smoke. When an oil breaks down under heat, the flavour of the oil shifts and toxic by-products such as transfats, aldehydes and lipid peroxides are produced. Heating for a long time encourages reactions with oxygen and the oil becomes oxidised and rancid.

Not only is the smoke point of extra virgin olive oil well above normal cooking temperatures, the smoke point is a rather inaccurate measurement of the stability of an oil. There is no single "point" at which the chemistry of an oil changes. Oxidation of an oil during heating is a more complex process. It is much more useful to talk about an oil's ability to resist oxidation. The three main factors that influence an oils oxidative stability are the level of naturally occurring antioxidants, the type of fats it contains and the method of processing and production. Experiments have compared the performance at high cooking temperatures for long periods of extra virgin olive oil with other cooking oils such as vegetable oils, seed oils including canola/rapeseed and coconut oil. The overall best performing oil in terms of antioxidant levels, stability and protection from the formation of transfats and other harmful compounds was extra virgin olive oil.

Longstanding advocates of the Mediterranean Diet advise that cooking destroys some of the antioxidants in extra virgin olive oil and so recommend the adding back of fresh oil for flavour, texture and antioxidants. Whilst this remains true, we are also understanding that the reduction in antioxidants of extra virgin olive oil during cooking occurs at the same time as the combining of antioxidants between foods which is very beneficial.

It seems that cooking with extra virgin olive oil is not only safe, but also desirable. The results of the antioxidant exchange between foods in the cooking process might be even more important than the effects of the antioxidants in the individual raw foods themselves.

Extra Virgin Olive Oil, Food Combinations and the Magic that Makes the Mediterranean Diet

The most exciting developments in our understanding of nutrition are in the fields of polyphenols and other plant "bioactive compounds", interactions within the food matrix and between ingredients in meals, and the influence of our gut microbes. This is why debates about macronutrients alone are so behind the curve. There are a number of particularly interesting discoveries which contribute significantly to the powerful effect of the Mediterranean Diet far beyond the consumption of the foods themselves. With this knowledge we have the key to unlock some of the greatest secrets of the diet and to truly access the unique health benefits. Here are some of the remarkable revelations that are not widely known but have important implications and tell us a great deal about the way the Mediterranean Diet with extra virgin olive oil exerts its effects.

For example, there is an exchange of polyphenols between vegetables and extra virgin olive oil when cooked together. The end result is a far greater abundance of these beneficial bioactive compounds available for absorption. The sum of health effects is greater than the individual ingredient parts. Researchers in Spain experimented by cooking eggplant, tomatoes, potatoes and pumpkin using different techniques. When cooked with extra virgin olive oil they showed that there was transfer of important olive oil polyphenols such as hydroxytyrosol and oleuropein into the vegetables. There was also movement the other way.

Vegetable polyphenols and carotenoid antioxidants such as beta-carotene and lycopene increased in the extra virgin olive oil coating the foods. Perhaps the most exciting finding has been the appearance of entirely new antioxidant polyphenols which were in neither the raw vegetables or the extra virgin olive oil at the beginning of the cooking, but were generated by the cooking process itself. This is the alchemy of the Mediterranean way of preparing foods together. Whether cooked in a tagine or simply roasted together, vegetables are invariably prepared and cooked in extra virgin olive oil in Mediterranean cuisine.

Adding extra virgin olive oil to carbohydrates has the dual effect of suppressing the speed at which the carbohydrate sugars are broken down, absorbed and released into the circulation as well as increasing insulin sensitivity. This reduction in glycaemic load of carbohydrates and refinement of the insulin response is probably one of the factors which makes a diet rich in extra virgin oil protective against both obesity and type 2 diabetes. It is unimaginable for someone in Italy to eat pasta without a drizzle of oil or for a visitor to be invited to share a traditional Middle Eastern flatbread or Greek pitta without the accompanying bottle of extra virgin olive oil.

It has been shown that the combination of the monounsaturated fats in extra virgin olive oil used as a dressing with nitrogen compounds in plants such as salads produce nitro fatty acids which, in synergy with polyphenols, lower blood pressure.

Healthy Omega 3 polyunsaturated fats in oily fish such as salmon, tuna, sea bass and bream are less tolerant of high temperatures than antioxidant rich monounsaturated extra virgin olive oil. When frying or baking fish in extra virgin olive oil, the omega 3s are coated and protected in the oil during heating and there is exchange of nutrients between fish and oil which results in the preservation and enriching of the precious omega 3 fats in the cooking juices.

As red meat is cooked it darkens in colour with the formation of heterocyclic amines and other compounds which have been implicated in causing cancers, especially bowel cancer. This may particularly be the case with barbequed meats. Marinating and cooking in an antioxidant rich mixture, for example with extra virgin olive oil, herbs, spices, garlic and red wine has been shown to decrease the formation of these compounds by as much as eighty percent. This is common practice in the Mediterranean where levels of cancer are very low.

Cooking healthy foods in extra virgin olive oil ensures that fat soluble nutrients are absorbed. Perhaps the best example of the importance of considering the impact of food combinations is the fact that a diet rich in extra virgin olive oil is associated with higher levels of Vitamin D – a vitamin which is important for many aspects of health including maintenance of bone strength and a healthy immune system. Extra virgin olive oil itself contains no Vitamin D. However through positive effects on the gut microbiome and by providing a vehicle for efficient absorption, it is particularly helpful in maximising the Vitamin D available to the body.

In many parts of the world the consumption of alcohol is associated with ill health and yet as part of the Mediterranean Diet, a glass or two of red wine (and to a lesser extent white wine) most days is believed to make a positive

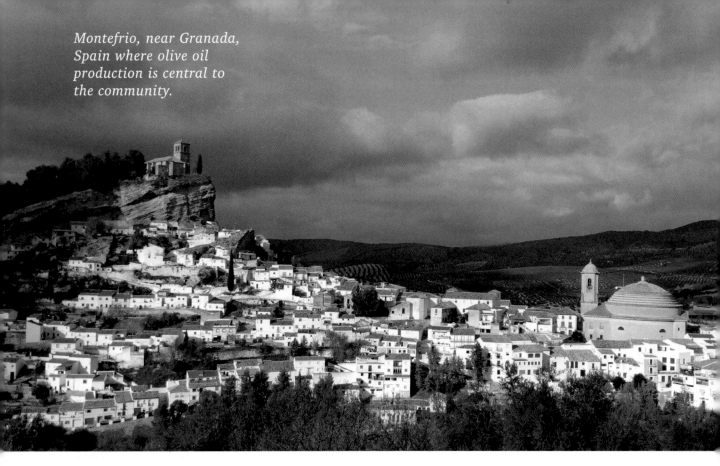

Montefrio, near Granada, Spain where olive oil production is central to the community.

contribution to longevity and reduce rates of heart disease and dementia. Drinking wine with a meal and in modest quantities rather than as part of a binge drinking culture is very clearly linked to slower absorption of alcohol and reduction in levels of toxic by-products such as acetaldehyde. It is likely that the benefits of the polyphenols in the wine, which have considerable potential antioxidant effects, can be enjoyed without the harm of peaks in blood alcohol levels. There is also research which confirms that the combination of extra virgin olive oil and red wine in a meal increased the availability of polyphenols from both the oil and the wine. The secret of healthy wine in the Mediterranean may be in its consumption with a meal rich in extra virgin olive oil.

Common Olive Oil Myths

There are many misconceptions about the Mediterranean Diet and especially extra virgin olive oil. It is time to debunk some of these myths.

The Mediterranean Diet is not just about eating more fruit and vegetables. It is not possible to take extra virgin olive oil out of the Diet. Other oils, even if they might contain healthy fats simply do not have the antioxidant capacity.

The fruit of the olive tree needs polyphenol protection from heat, light and oxygen in its dynamic interaction with the environment much more than the relatively inert seeds from which some other oils are made.

It is the antioxidant capacity which protects extra virgin olive oil and makes it the healthiest oil with which to cook. It is important to use good quality oil for cooking.

Some myths surround the modest percentage of saturated fat in extra virgin olive oil. Not only is it a relatively small amount but there is no evidence that the particular saturated fats adversely affect cholesterol levels. There are differences in saturated fats, including how they are absorbed and extra virgin olive oil has been shown to consistently not only benefit cholesterol levels, but perhaps more importantly reduce the levels of harmful oxidation of cholesterol.

Extra virgin olive oil is of course mainly comprised of fat, though it is as a vehicle for the "minor constituents" such as polyphenols that it is probably most beneficial as a food. Fats contain more calories than carbohydrates and proteins. However, it is a myth that extra virgin olive oil, as part of a Mediterranean way of eating, is fattening. Weight gain, obesity and diabetes are not simply a consequence of calorie intake. It is more about portion size, satiety, meal constituents, type of fats eaten and the glycaemic load of meals.

There are claims that extra virgin olive oil is expensive. This is, of course, relative, and depends on what a consumer judges to be good value. It is so essential to the Mediterranean Diet, and is such a healthy and versatile unrefined fresh fruit juice that it is no wonder it costs more to produce. The investment needed to nurture trees, individually harvest by hand or machine, press and carefully store and transport is much more than that associated with more industrial methods of seed or vegetable oil production.

Yet it is possible to purchase a month's worth of excellent quality oil for everyday use and for the table, perhaps in tins or a box (which is incidentally a good packageing system for preservation of antioxidants) for the price of a couple of cups of latte in a favourite coffee shop. As the value of extra virgin olive oil becomes apparent, it is clear that this is a choice which can be made, just as a choice can be made to buy a bottle of wine for an evening or to spend money on a take away meal. Just as there are fine wines, so there are also fine extra virgin olive oils. It is again a choice which can be made to buy such oils for even more flavour and enjoyment.

Whilst it is possible to buy excellent oils within a reasonable budget, given the cost of production and assuming the consumer is willing to spend a minimum amount to ensure quality, it is certainly not the case that all extra virgin olive oils are the same. Some are relatively sweet and mild in flavour whilst others are more robust and pungent. Each oil has its own unique aroma and taste profile and this will vary from year to year. It is remarkable that the flavour of each oil tells a story of the year experienced by the tree – the winter frosts, perhaps Mistral winds sweeping south across the Mediterranean and the intensity of the summer's heat. This is a unique and extraordinary food.

There have been several articles in the media suggesting that there is a lot of fake extra virgin olive oil around. These days the olive oil industry is one of the most closely regulated in the world, and as long as it is bought from a reputable producer and supplier consumers can be very reassured that they will be buying a high-quality product. Freshness and the conditions of storage are extremely important to ensure the sensory and chemical parameters of extra virginity are maintained, and so any oil which has been mishandled or is getting close to its "best before" date may have deteriorated. It is important to understand how to select the best oils.

How to Choose the Best – A Buyer's Guide

When it comes to choosing an extra virgin olive oil, some people might buy one for everyday use in cooking and food preparation and another, finer oil, for "anointing" or finishing a dish. This is not necessary if you have a good quality extra virgin olive oil in larger containers and instead smaller amounts can be decanted into a bottle for the table. It is entirely a matter of taste and economy. But there are some guiding principles which are important for making the right choice.

Fresh oil is best. Polyphenol levels reduce over time as extra virgin olive oil is gradually oxidised – eventually to the point of rancidity. Health benefits diminish, with polyphenols halving, on average, over twelve months. Producers now often place on label a harvest date as well as a "best before" date. The "best before" date may be eighteen months from time of bottling which in turn may occur following time stored in stainless steel containers under liquid nitrogen to exclude oxygen at the mill. So, it is best to buy the most recently harvested oil. Harvest times range in general from September to January in the Northern Hemisphere; April,

May and June are common months to harvest in the Southern hemisphere such as Australia and South America. Some oils are produced on a family estate, others may be from a mill owned by a cooperative. Some are blends of oils from many countries. Given that quality relates to the careful and quick harvesting, transfer, pressing and storage of extra virgin olive oil, it is reasonable to expect that the more local oils will be better. Growers are in general fiercely proud of their hard work in producing excellence in oils and it is understandable that they try to communicate this in their marketing.

Acidity may be quoted on the label, the lower the better. And polyphenols may also be measured.

There is no "right" level of polyphenols, however total polyphenols in oils measured above 250mg/kg are known have positive health benefits. Many, but not all oils will achieve this and in particular oils which are purposely blended to have a bland taste, which some consumers are said to like, may fall below this. Peppery oils have excellent polyphenol levels of between 300 and 800 mg/kg and producers can achieve harmony of flavour with some bitterness and pungency combined with attractive fruitiness and other notes. A few oils have even higher levels into the thousands and may be marketed as supplements rather than food. Some of the research studies which show extra virgin olive oil contributing to reduced inflammatory markers, oxidative stress and even end points such as reduced risk of heart disease, stroke, cancers and death have specifically used high polyphenol oils, though always oils consumed as food rather than supplements. Compliance with the Mediterranean Diet has been measured by the presence of polyphenols in the study participants' urine, showing the significance attached to these dietary compounds specific to extra virgin olive oil in such research.

However, given the variation in consumption of oils, there is no doubt that we should celebrate good quality sweet and mild oils as well as higher polyphenol pungent or bitter oils and enjoy them as food with different dishes, and so long as we have a quantity of oil consistent with the Mediterranean Diet, we can safely assume the health benefits will be achieved.

Tasting notes may be available on the labels of oils. The more robust or peppery an oil, the higher the likely levels of polyphenols.

Extra virgin olive oil is best stored free of oxygen, heat and light. A dark bottle or container will help preserve the oil. A vacuum-sealed foil bag in a box preserves oil even better and some producers have started to use these especially for 3- and 5-litre quantities.

Summary

Extra virgin olive oil, uniquely among foods, has extensive and measurable benefits on health.

Two or three tablespoonfuls of extra virgin olive oil each day contributes significantly and inseparably to the Mediterranean Diet.

Extraordinary polyphenols in extra virgin olive oil are influenced by origin and methods of production.

Combining ingredients with extra virgin olive oil in preparation and cooking creates powerful added synergistic health benefits.

It is possible to taste the health in the fruitiness, bitterness and peppery flavours of extra virgin olive oil.

Chapter Seven

Foods of the Mediterranean Diet

"I went out into the garden in the morning dusk, when sorrow enveloped me like a cloud; And the breeze brought to my nostril the odour of spices, as balm of healing for a sick soul."
Moses ibn Ezra

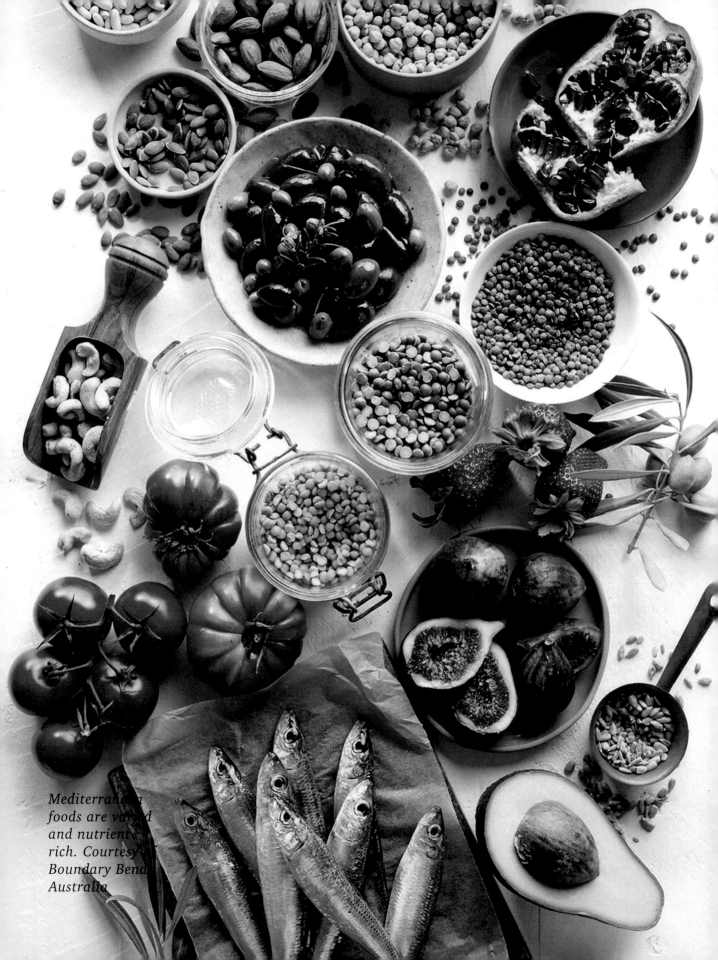

Mediterranean foods are varied and nutrient rich. Courtesy of Boundary Bend, Australia

Macronutrients in 30 Seconds – Carbs, Fats and Proteins

Most of the nutrients we consume are in the form of the big three macronutrients so familiar to us because they are the subject of so much debate about how much or little of each we should consume.

Carbohydrates are a source of energy. They can exist in slowly absorbed forms such as fibrous wholegrains, or more simple forms such as corn syrup in many processed foods which are likely to cause harmful spikes in blood sugars. Fats, of which there are many types, are a denser source of calories and are also important for cell structure. Proteins are often characterized as the building block molecules of life. The Mediterranean Diet when described in the simplest of ways provides a perfect balance of high fibre and low glycaemic index carbohydrates, healthy fat combinations and proteins derived mainly from plants such as beans, nuts and fish rather than large and frequent portions of red meat.

Micronutrients in 30 seconds – Vitamins, Minerals and Bioactive Polyphenols

The micronutrient content of foods is what really matters in delivering the powerful effects of the real Mediterranean Diet.

Vitamins are essential nutrients which are unable to be made by the body. They are involved in a number of important functions in growth and maintenance of health.

Minerals such as zinc, selenium, calcium and potassium have numerous roles from ensuring bone strength, blood pressure control and heart rhythm through to hormone regulation, chemical messageing in cells, DNA function and cell division.

The many thousands of plant bioactive compounds, including polyphenols so abundant in the Mediterranean Diet are being researched for their potential antioxidant, anti-inflammatory and cancer preventing properties which may contribute to the decreased rates of chronic disease including heart disease, cancers and dementia associated with the diet. It is a mistake to focus entirely on the three hundred grams of carbohydrate or fifty grams of fat and protein an average person might consume each day whilst ignoring the disproportionate positive power of the single gram of polyphenols.

All the Superfoods you can think of?

It is helpful to think about the many ingredients of the Mediterranean Diet with a degree of flexibility. Foods can be added from other food cultures and contribute to the healthiest diet in the world. A list of common constituents can be used to show the variety of readily available foods that can be incorporated into a weekly shopping trip and included in recipes or prepared with extra virgin olive oil as part of a simple dish.

The term "superfood" has been used for marketing specific nutrient rich foods. There is, however, no definition of a superfood, and they often seem to be individual foods which are normally consumed in relatively small amounts in a diet. It would be misleading to claim that rare green algae for example had miraculous healing effects. There might also be significant environmental costs of shipping large quantities of Himalayan berries simply because there has been excitement whipped up in a magazine article. A food producer might have a novel idea of creating a potato chip incorporating kale yet it might be heavily salted and created using unhealthy oils. The antioxidant carotenoid compound called lutein found in natural kale, which might be singled out for praise, will be vastly depleted in such processing. Lutein from sources such as kale is much more readily absorbed as part of a Mediterranean style meal, rich in other healthy nutrients with synergistic effects, and supportive of the diverse gut microbiome needed to enjoy its benefits.

Many of the foods of the Mediterranean Diet could be regarded as superfoods. However, it is the bringing of them together which supercharges the effects of the micronutrients and bioactive compounds within them.

Foods of the Mediterranean Diet – Colourful Vegetables

Vegetables, when combined with extra virgin olive oil are the foundation of the Mediterranean Diet. They are a source of low GI carbohydrate, fibre, vitamins, minerals and various combinations of the thousands of polyphenols and carotenoids which often give them colour and add to their taste. Compounds such as lignans, flavanols, anthocyanins, catechins, quercetin, phenolic acids and stilbenes may one day become familiar names to us as we learn more about their anti-inflammatory, antioxidant and anti-cancer effects as well as early signs that many support a healthy immune function.

Common vegetables of the Mediterranean Diet include:
artichokes, asparagus, aubergine (eggplant), beetroot, bell peppers, broccoli, brussels sprouts, cabbage, carrots, celery, celeriac, chicory, courgettes (zucchini), cucumbers, fennel, greens, kale, leeks, lettuce, mushrooms, okra, onions, potatoes, pumpkin, purslane, radishes, shallots, spinach, sweet potatoes, tomatoes (really a fruit, but mostly used as a vegetable) and turnips.

Foods of the Mediterranean Diet – Fruits

With a much lower GI profile than the juices we frequently consume, whole fruits of the Mediterranean Diet are rich in fibre and are an excellent source of vitamin C in particular. Their outer skins are often the greatest source of polyphenols and carotenoids providing the reds, blues, purples and oranges which are so plentiful on a Mediterranean plate.

Common Fruits of the Mediterranean Diet include:
apples, apricots, avocados (often used in savoury dishes rather than as a fruit), blackberries, blueberries, cherries, clementines, dates, figs, grapefruits, grapes, lemons, melons, nectarines, olives, oranges, peaches, pears, pomegranates, raspberries, strawberries and tangerines.

Foods of the Mediterranean Diet – Wholegrains

Wholegrains are cereals which have their outer husk intact. This increases the amount of fibre, reduces the glycaemic index and it is also the husk where many of the vitamins, minerals and protective polyphenols of the grain are concentrated. Wholegrain rice, breads and pasta preserve these nutritional advantages in contrast to processed white rice and breads for example.

The methods of production of wholegrains further influence their value. Modern wheat has been selectively bred to be uniform in height and structure to make industrial farming easier. Unfortunately, the loss of diversity has also resulted in a reduction in mineral and polyphenol content as well as an increase in gluten. This is why older varieties of cereals have become more popular, though the consumption of these "ancient grains" still remains a tiny fraction overall. There has also been a renaissance of older styles of baking such as using a sourdough starter because the glycaemic index may be lower.

Common wholegrains of the Mediterranean Diet include:
barley, buckwheat, bulgar, farro, millet, oats, polenta, rice, rye, spelt and wheat

Foods of the Mediterranean Diet – Beans, Peas and Lentils (Legumes and Pulses)

This is a section about legumes, but many people are not familiar with the word. It describes a plant with a pod with seeds within. Sometimes the pod itself is edible, for example, with French beans or mangetout (the French very practically name this pea "eat everything" in case it was not obvious). The contents of the pod whether it be bean, pea or lentil are collectively known as pulses.

Pulses are consumed in much higher quantities in the Mediterranean than other parts of the world, and are a common ingredient in an extra virgin olive oil rich casserole for example. Pulses are a generous package of protein, fibre, vitamins, minerals and polyphenols and are consumed several times a week. Some need soaking overnight to soften them before cooking. This may be perceived as a barrier to their use although it is well worth the wait when they are combined with other ingredients in a warm winter stew. Alternatively, prepared beans can be bought in cans or soaked and then frozen. Lentils on the other hand can be cooked without prior soaking – in stews or, for example, added to a sofrito type of dish to simmer with fried onions, other vegetables and chopped tomatoes or passata.

Common legumes of the Mediterranean Diet include:
cannellini beans, chickpeas, fava (broad) beans, French beans, gigantes beans, green beans, kidney beans, lentils, mangetout, peas and split peas.

Foods of the Mediterranean Diet – Nuts and Seeds

Nuts are a common staple of the Mediterranean Diet and are a powerhouse of good fats, B and E vitamins, abundant polyphenols and minerals like calcium, iron, zinc, potassium, magnesium, selenium, manganese and copper which play such an important role in health. Studies have shown the benefits for heart health of a handful (30g) of unsalted nuts each day. Seeds also provide a great source of healthy fats and minerals.

Common nuts and seeds of the Mediterranean Diet include:
almonds, cashews, flax seeds, hazelnuts, pine nuts, pistachios, pumpkin seeds, sesame seeds and walnuts.

Foods of the Mediterranean Diet – Herbs and Spices

Herbs and spices are a concentration of bioactive compounds, including polyphenols, many of which are quite specific to the individual plant. They have high antioxidant capacity and individual spices may have measurable anti-inflammatory effects. Turmeric has been studied for its possible benefits when used as an adjunct to therapies for bowel cancer, rosemary has been cited as a contributing factor to the longevity of the inhabitants of southern Italy and the inclusion of chilli a few times a week has been shown to be associated with a reduced risk of heart disease. An active component of chilli known as capsaicin can be used for pain relief in a commercially available cream.

Spice combinations such as those in za'atar and harissa are common in the cuisines of the Middle East and North Africa, giving particular tastes to familiar dishes. Garlic is in the same family as onions. It is more commonly regarded as a spice than a vegetable, though the distinction is rather arbitrary. Garlic contains antioxidant compounds called allicins, which may be helpful for blood pressure, immunity and decrease the risk of blood clots. Sometimes the spices may be the seed of the plant such as cumin, mustard or fennel. Fennel plant is often regarded as a vegetable, its seeds as a spice. Many spices are derived from the bark or root of a plant such as ginger and cinnamon, whereas basil and rosemary are examples of leaves.

Common herbs and spices in the Mediterranean Diet include:
basil, bay leaf, chillies, cinnamon, cloves, cumin, fennel, garlic, ginger, marjoram, mint, oregano, parsley, pepper, rosemary, sage, star anise, sumac, tarragon, thyme and turmeric.

Foods of the Mediterranean Diet – Dairy

Dairy products feature in modest amounts each day in a typical Mediterranean Diet. Dietary advice in other parts of the world has recommended a reduction in consumption due to the saturated fat content. One unfortunate consequence of this has been the proliferation of high sugar flavoured low fat yoghurts.

The truth is that the dairy foods consumed in the Mediterranean region are typically fermented products – unprocessed cheeses and yoghurts from the milk of sheep and goats. There is no convincing evidence that such food in modest amounts should be avoided. In fact, their daily consumption has been shown to not only provide healthy sources of calcium, but also create a vibrant and diverse gut microbiome and reduce the risk of developing diabetes.

It is important to note that some products, for example "Greek yoghurt" which traditionally were made from the milk of sheep or goats have been adapted and now are frequently comprised of cow's milk. The nutritional profile will be changed.

Common dairy products in the Mediterranean Diet include:
feta, haloumi, manchego, kefir (a yoghurt type of drink), Parmigiano-Reggiano, pecorino, ricotta and yogurt (including Greek yogurt).

It is a real pleasure to be able to observe that there are thousands of cheese varieties native to the Mediterranean and it is impossible for a list such as this to do justice to the breadth of flavour and production methods of artisanal cheeses of the region.

Foods of the Mediterranean Diet – Seafood

Seafood was consumed regularly in the coastal areas of the Mediterranean, perhaps as frequently as two or three times a week. In contrast there would have been less reliance on fish by communities in the interior of countries bordering the sea. Seafood is a particularly important source of lean protein, vitamins and minerals as well as omega 3 fats which may have anti-inflammatory effects and possibly provide protection from heart disease. It should be noted that there are some concerns about the concentration of pollutant heavy metals such as mercury in the largest fish of the food chain and also legitimate worries about sustainability. Alternative sources of omega 3 fats for vegetarian diets include nuts, seeds and some green leafy vegetables.

Common seafood in the Mediterranean Diet includes:
anchovies, cod, clams, cockles, crab, eel, flounder, lobster, mackerel, mussels, octopus, oysters, prawns, salmon, sardines, sea bass, sea bream, shrimp, squid, swordfish, trout, tuna and whitebait.

Foods of the Mediterranean Diet – Meat

Meat, especially red meat, is less commonly consumed than in other countries and is served in smaller quantities. Here it is very important to stress the description of the traditional diet. Meat consumption in the region has increased in modern times.

Chicken is perhaps the commonest meat in the Mediterranean Diet. Wild game birds such as partridge also appear in older recipes. Chicken is easy to rear and provides healthy, lean meat. Eggs are a good source of protein and vitamin D.

Lamb, goat or pork were eaten on feast days in more affluent households. Anyone who has lived in the Mediterranean will understand that there are often Saints' Days and other regular festivals but the slaughter and consumption of red meat would have been limited to perhaps once a fortnight or once a month at the most. Quantities would have been modest and every part of the animal would have been used to feed the extended family. Rabbit is a meat rarely eaten in other parts of the world but was often a more affordable option. Beef was not generally consumed in the traditional Mediterranean Diet.

The quality of the meat in the diet was very different to the majority of meat reared with modern methods of animal husbandry. All animals would be naturally forageing and free range, getting plenty of space to roam and explore a varied diet. This has measurable and demonstrable effects on the leanness and proportions of fats in the meat.

When it comes to meat, it is important to ask what your food ate. And indeed, how the animals are raised in general. This makes a difference not only to the quality of life of the animal but also to the quality of food produced in nutrition as well as taste. Animals bred, housed and fed intensively will make cheaper but much poorer quality meat. If it costs a little more, then the simple answer is to enjoy it in smaller portions, complimenting the rich flavours of high-quality meat with many more interesting accompanying vegetables.

An example of this is in Iberico pork. Raised with freedom in Southern Spain and Portugal to search out their favorite diet of acorns, the meat not only looks different but also has a rich and nutty flavour. Remarkably, more than fifty percent of the fat is healthy monounsaturated – that is the same fat that is found in nuts and olive oil. This is the kind of meat our ancestors would have hunted.

Preserved meats are a subject of controversy. Processed meats are likely to contribute to a higher risk of cancer. It is possible that this association relates to the sodium nitrite used as a preservative to prevent food borne illnesses from contamination. Some regions have resisted the need to add preservatives other than salt to hams and salami and with assurances of safe methods of production traditional products like Parma ham may be nitrite free.

Foods of the Mediterranean Diet – Miscellaneous

Chocolate is a relatively recent addition to the Mediterranean Diet, having been brought back from the Americas by Columbus and introduced to the Spanish court. The indigenous peoples of Mexico valued the drink made from the cacao tree bean as a medicine, believing the bitterest chocolate to relieve stomach complaints. The sweetened, sugary chocolate with a low percentage of cocoa is much less healthy than the more bitter, high antioxidant high percentage chocolate. Acquiring the taste by graduating from seventy percent cocoa chocolate through to a small square of ninety percent each day is a worthwhile journey.

In general the higher the percentage of cocoa the higher the levels of flavonoid polyphenol antioxidants and the lower the proportion of sugars, although different brands of the same grade of chocolate may vary considerably in the amount of sugar. It is always worth reading the label.

Honey is the natural sweetener of the Mediterranean Diet, though not suitable for infant diets. Although it is high in sugars, the quantity and way in which it is consumed in the Mediterranean is not thought to contribute towards obesity or to be pro-inflammatory. In fact, the reverse is the case. The natural antibacterial compounds and antioxidant polyphenols are beneficial for health. These are lowered by heating processes which are applied to many commercial honeys. "Raw" honeys retain more polyphenols than treated honeys which are most frequently sold in supermarkets. The nectar and pollen forage sources of bees makes a difference to the taste of the honey but there is currently insufficient research to draw conclusions about whether nutritional effects are different between for example thyme, lavender or pine and fir tree honeys.

Vinegars are a common condiment in the Mediterranean Diet. The astringent or tart taste compliments many dishes. There are many claims about benefits of vinegars, a number of which are not substantiated by robust evidence. However, it certainly seems to be the case that vinegars may improve blood sugar levels after a meal. Balsamic vinegar is worthy of a special mention. As with so many foods this can vary enormously in quality. Cheap balsamic vinegars may have been sweetened artificially with caramel, but the authentic aged fermented grape juice using traditional methods will have a naturally perfect balance of sweetness and tartness and will be rich in polyphenols. Balsamic vinegar can be enjoyed on grilled meats or fish, with salads or even with fruit or cheese.

Snails are an irresistible addition to this section. They are often associated with French cuisine but have been farmed or collected from the wild on the Greek islands for centuries. During some periods of history, they have contributed significantly as a source of protein as well as adding vitamins and minerals to the diet.

Beverages in the Mediterranean Diet

Water is the commonest beverage in the Mediterranean Diet. There is no tradition for high sugar and sodium sodas or carbonated drinks. Water can be flavoured with a little fresh lemon or lime juice.

Wine is commonly drunk with a meal in many parts of the Mediterranean though religious observance requires abstinence from alcohol in some regions. Both red and white wines are enjoyed, but it is the polyphenols called procyanidins and resveratrol from the red grape skin which have been of particular interest in terms of possible health benefits. The anti-inflammatory and antioxidant effects have been linked to reduced risks of heart disease and blood clots. Although champagne is light in colour it is made from a combination of grapes including the red and black varieties of pinot noir and pinot meunier and has higher levels of polyphenols than sparkling wines which use only white grapes.

In general, wine has increased in alcohol content in recent years and quality has often been associated with softer, aged wines. In fact, these are likely to be lower in antioxidants than younger wines with a more robust taste. The "laying down" of wines was not a feature of the more traditional Mediterranean Diet, where country wines of the most recent season were an accompaniment to a meal.

There are a number of factors which affect the polyphenol content of wine including the fermentation process, how much the skin has been involved in its production and the maceration time as well as the variety and the conditions of growth of the vines. The availability of the polyphenols, as well as a reduction in the negative effect of alcohol is affected by the meal with which wine is drunk. Some parallels can be drawn with extra virgin olive oil in terms of what might predict high polyphenol levels. Just as some olive varieties are naturally rich in polyphenols, wine from the tannat and malbec grapes of South West France or South America and the cannonau wines of Sardinia grown at some altitude from older vines may have higher levels of procyanidin polyphenols. There have been large studies linking alcohol consumption with cancer and earlier death, however it is very likely that moderate wine consumption in the style of the Mediterranean Diet is good for health. The benefits for this subgroup of drinkers may well be lost amongst the statistical "noise" of the unhealthy habits of binge drinking, riskier behaviour among some groups, overconsumption and the different types of alcoholic drink included in such studies.

Teas are a longstanding part of the Mediterranean Diet and predate the introduction of coffee. There are many types of herbal teas available in the Mediterranean. Herbs and spices can be infused with hot water and enjoyed at any time of the day. Mint tea is a particular favorite in Turkey and the Near East, with sage tea and Greek mountain tea amongst those consumed in Greece. There are mixtures of herbs and spices which have been adopted by particular populations and made their own, for example "Bedouin Tea" being a mix of black tea, dried rosebuds and cinnamon. Herbs and spices contain many antioxidant polyphenols.

Drinking the brew from roasted coffee beans brought from Ethiopia is thought to have been conceived in Arabia in the fifteenth century. From these beginnings it spread across North Africa and into the European countries of the Mediterranean. There are numerous antioxidant polyphenols in coffee which have been associated with health benefits. Coffee also contains caffeine which is a stimulant, may have mild addictive properties and can if consumed in excess affect susceptible individuals by increasing heart rate and levels of anxiety. However, a moderate intake can be part of the Mediterranean Diet.

Mediterranean Diet Pyramid

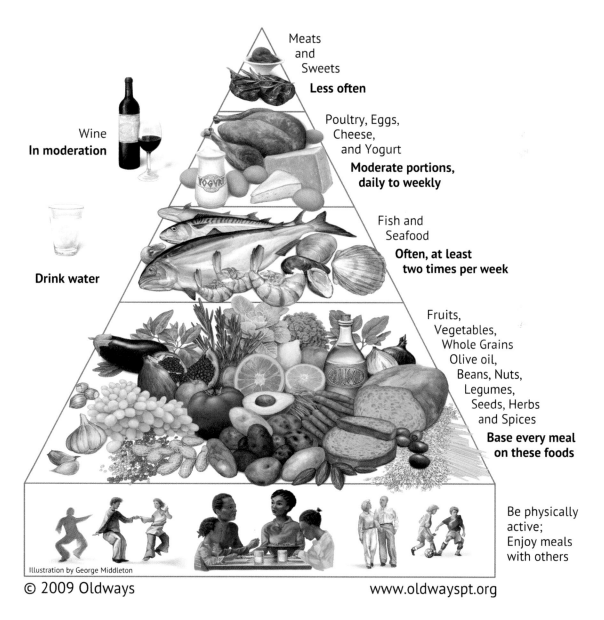

Meats
and
Sweets
Less often

Wine
In moderation

Poultry, Eggs,
Cheese,
and Yogurt
**Moderate portions,
daily to weekly**

Fish and
Seafood
**Often, at least
two times per week**

Drink water

Fruits,
Vegetables,
Whole Grains
Olive oil,
Beans, Nuts,
Legumes,
Seeds, Herbs
and Spices
**Base every meal
on these foods**

Be physically
active;
Enjoy meals
with others

Illustration by George Middleton

© 2009 Oldways

www.oldwayspt.org

Reproduced by kind permission of Oldways

Summary

The Mediterranean Diet ticks the basic nutritional boxes for good health.

The Mediterranean Diet is a rich anti-inflammatory high polyphenol diet.

There are specific reasons why the ingredients in the diet promote health.

The combination of foods together results in the gold standard healthy diet.

Beverages are included in the diet and confer health.

Chapter Eight

Eating to Save the Planet

"A society grows great when its elders plant trees under whose shade they know they will never sit."
Greek Proverb

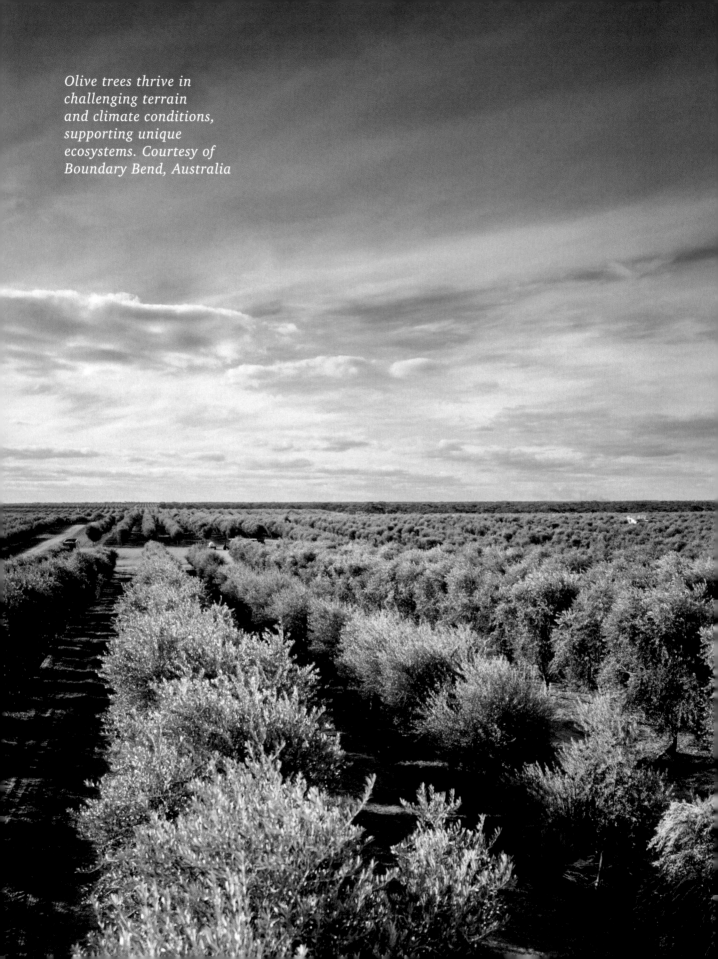

Olive trees thrive in challenging terrain and climate conditions, supporting unique ecosystems. Courtesy of Boundary Bend, Australia

The Sustainable Mediterranean Diet

Agriculture and food supply contribute significantly to the production of greenhouse gases. At the time of writing this is thought to be as much as thirty percent, more than the effects of planes, trains and automobiles.

The rearing of meat is a particular problem since methane gas produced by herbivores, especially cattle raised for beef, does significant damage to the environment. Cows are not a common sight in the Mediterranean. Dairy and meat produce, when they are eaten, are mainly from smaller livestock such as sheep, goat or pigs which contribute considerably less to emissions, and of course the addition of extra virgin olive oil can enhance and encourage consumption of locally-produced seasonal vegetables anywhere in the world.

The wealthier countries of the world have an apparently insatiable appetite for red meat. A shift to a more plant predominant diet would not only decrease greenhouse gas emissions but would also be more likely to be able to feed the population of our planet since there is greater yield of plant than animal food per hectare.

The mass produced, poor quality, intensively farmed meat we consume in such large quantities in western diets is accelerating the climate crisis.

The traditional Mediterranean Diet is often cited as a sustainable diet, in contrast with the diets of the modern world. The quantity of red meat consumed in the traditional Mediterranean Diet is very modest, and in general this was the preserve of holidays and festivals. The quality of meat would tend to be higher – leaner and more naturally fed. Thomas Jefferson, the founding father foodie president of the USA and an advocate of the Mediterranean Diet long before the term was coined and recognised for its health benefits, regarded meat as a condiment to his meals which were primarily of vegetables.

A publication in Spain mapped the likely environmental outcome of different dietary patterns. A more Western diet was predicted to increase factors harmful for the environment by as much as 72%, whilst a shift towards a more Mediterranean diet would reduce greenhouse gas emissions by 70%, energy consumption by 52% and water consumption by 33%.

The combination of wholegrains, vegetables and extra virgin olive oil with modest quantities of cheese and yoghurt from sheep and goats is a sustainable dietary model. Many countries are able to produce their own extra virgin olive oil and there are groves being planted in new regions all the time. Transportation of extra virgin olive oil to cooler climates is a necessary part of exporting the benefits of the diet, and of course it is compatible with locally produced seasonal vegetables anywhere in the world. Planting olive trees improves soil quality, requires relatively low water usage, decreases desertification, and preserves and encourages biodiversity. An olive grove, well managed, creates its own ecosystem and sustains a wide variety of species. In the production of one litre of extra virgin olive oil, ten kilograms of carbon dioxide is removed from the atmosphere. The olive tree "sinks" carbon and with best agricultural practices this can mean ten tonnes of carbon dioxide per hectare per year can be "fixed" as a positive contribution to reversing the risk of climate change. As its use in food preparation enhances the palatability of vegetables and it is the foundation of the plant-based Mediterranean Diet, the contribution of extra virgin olive oil in mitigating climate change needs to be particularly acknowledged.

With increasing demand for seafood, it is important that fish is consumed in a way that is sustainable. There are some fish reserves which are becoming depleted and this can vary from region to region and also depend on fishing methods. There is now reliable information available on the Internet which describes which fish are at most risk of overconsumption.

The traditional Mediterranean Diet was a diet typically consumed by people of the region who were farmers or labourers. Food was valued not only for its nourishment and enjoyment but also because there were times when food was scarce. Wastage was therefore kept to an absolute minimum and ingenious ways of using "leftovers" were employed to ensure that the most benefit was gained from a meal. Many dishes of the Mediterranean Diet are suitable for storage or use ingredients which lend themselves to safely be "recycled" to a further meal. The amount of food discarded was minimal out of necessity in comparison with modern ways of life. Lessons in sustainability can be learned from the respect for the value of food in the Mediterranean Diet.

Summary

The meat and dairy industry contribute significantly to greenhouse gas production – cows are the main offenders.

The Mediterranean Diet, being plant predominant, is an environmentally friendly diet.

The Mediterranean Diet relies largely on local, seasonal foods.

Consumption of extra virgin olive oil encourages a plant-based diet and the tree gives back to the environment.

Extra virgin olive oil is becoming a local product in many more parts of the world.

Chapter Nine

Bringing the Mediterranean Diet Home

"I have not told half of what I saw."
Marco Polo

Beyond the Mediterranean Shores

The Mediterranean Diet has evolved over millennia. The lands surrounding the Mediterranean Sea where the olive tree grows have been a place of trade and commerce throughout history, bringing new foods to the region and adding flavour and nutritional benefits to the diet.

Similarly, the ingredients of the region have been exported to new continents and the traditional cuisine of the Mediterranean has been embraced in many other parts of the world.

Franciscan monks and pioneering settlers introduced vineyards and olive groves to areas of the New World in both the Northern and Southern Hemispheres. Flavours brought by the Cajun peoples to Louisiana from Canada in the 18th Century were ultimately rooted in the origins of the first migration from France. In more recent times we have seen Italian immigration popularising many of the iconic dishes of the Mediterranean in cities in the USA and Australia. There are numerous examples of the dissemination of Mediterranean recipes and ways of preparing food.

Keeping the Truths Abroad

However, we must be cautious about believing that modern versions of Mediterranean dishes are always representative of the traditional Mediterranean Diet. There are many problems with this.

For example, the manufacture of pizza bought in take away restaurants or in the supermarket is very different from the traditional flatbread with tomato and herbs. Pizza has largely become a highly processed food.

Many "Mediterranean" restaurants use cheap vegetable oil for cooking and have poor quality olive oils for the table. The people of the Mediterranean themselves often abandon their traditional way of life and adopt western habits of eating.

Oils other than extra virgin olive oil are promoted as providing the same health benefits, or even claimed to have more healthy profiles. Canola oil, known as rapeseed oil in the UK has been advertised as a similarly monounsaturated fat predominant oil, but with "lower levels of saturated fat than olive oil". In such promotions it is not mentioned that the levels of saturated fat are low in both oils in the first place and that there is no evidence that the form of plant-based saturated fat in olive oil has any detrimental effect. Some rapeseed oil is described as "cold pressed" or "extra virgin" in an unregulated attempt to emulate the criteria of standards set for extra virgin olive oil. There is often the inevitable claim of a higher "smoke point", despite evidence that this does not accurately reflect the behaviour of oils when used in cooking. No reference is made to polyphenols or the science which shows extra virgin olive oil to be an intrinsic part of the Mediterranean Diet. It is simply not appropriate for marketeers to make comparisons with the pressed oil from the olive fruit which is inseparably at the heart of the Mediterranean Diet. Most seed oils or vegetable oils are created using industrial methods of production at high temperatures and with the use of solvents such as hexane.

The Mediterranean Diet can also be misappropriated by combatants in the various food fights which seem to attract so much controversial publicity. For example, those advocating the revision of the current guideline position on saturated fats reinvent the Mediterranean Diet with coconut oil or the regular use of butter. Many who denounce vegetarianism visit the Mediterranean and go in search of dishes of red meat which restaurants or hosts will gladly serve. Somehow it is then claimed, despite Mediterranean Diet Adherence Score evidence to the contrary, that red meat is an intrinsic part of daily life rather than an occasional addition to a plant predominant diet.

There is a story told in Nicotera describing Ancel Key's request to experience a typical meal of Southern Italy in the kitchen of a family employed in agricultural work. The hosting family, showing typical Calabrian pride and hospitality quietly negotiated with a neighbour to spend more than a week's wages on the purchase and slaughter of a goat. Dr Keys and his colleagues soon realised that the goat stew and other delicacies using every part of the animal were a celebration of their visit and a mark of generosity rather than the typical fare of "cucina povera" – the simple rustic, vegetable predominant cooking of the rural workers.

Heritage Diets and Health

This book is dedicated to the Mediterranean Diet, the subtleties of which rarely make the headlines but make all the difference to its potential for powerful and life changing effects.

There are of course other traditional diets which have been cited for their benefits. Elements of cuisines from many parts of the world have been investigated to establish the reasons for pockets of good population health. Whether it is the seafood or mushrooms of Japan, the beans of Costa Rica, the vegetarian diet of Seventh Day Adventist communities in California, the spices found in some Asian dishes or the tubers of Western Africa, food and nutrition will always be the subject of interest and research to find healthy ways of life.

On the other hand, many parts of the world are seeing unhealthy eating habits increase with soaring rates of obesity, diabetes and chronic diseases associated with chronic inflammation.

As we learn more about other diets, the story of amalgamating beneficial dietary traditions and exploring new ways to prepare and enjoy food can continue to be written. It is possible to combine the anti-inflammatory foods of many different cultures to reverse the impact and cost of the increasing burden of poor health described by the World Health Organisation.

As awareness of the Mediterranean Diet increases many countries are seeing an expansion in demand for extra virgin olive oil, met by increasing imports or, where the climate allows, the introduction of an olive oil industry of their own. People across the world are showing more interest in aligning their diets with the principles of the Mediterranean Diet. There is olive oil production in North and South America, Europe and Asia stretching from the birthplace of olive tree domestication in the Near East to India, China and Japan. North African olive oil cultivation on the Mediterranean coastline was established prior to the Greek and Roman empires and the regions of South Africa famous for wine production are now also becoming known for producing high quality extra virgin olive oil.

There is a need to improve understanding of the more nuanced aspects of diet, including the importance of food preparation and combinations for health, so that when diets are assimilated the advantages can be truly realised.

"Mediterraneanising" our Diets

Those of us in Northern Europe can use berries native to our climate in place of citrus fruits and incorporate them in a Mediterranean style diet. Although oats probably originated in the fertile crescent of the Near East, they are particularly well suited to wetter climates and so are more typically eaten in Northern Europe and contain many beneficial nutrients. Recipes with oats, extra virgin olive oil and honey are a delightful way to combine these ingredients from north and south. Rye bread adorned with pickled fish, tomatoes, dill and extra virgin olive oil incorporates these different culinary traditions. Cabbage, root vegetables and brussels sprouts roasted in extra virgin olive oil with onions and bell peppers is a similarly healthy coalescence of diverse native foods.

American cooking has been influenced by settlers from other countries, including from Southern Europe. Beans are used frequently in the Mediterranean Diet, perhaps twice a week or more and are also a staple of America. Squashes, avocados, cassava and sweet potatoes also lend themselves well to adaption and adoption, integrating local ingredients and common themes of the Mediterranean Diet. Pastry from anywhere in the world can be prepared more healthily using extra virgin olive oil.

Asian and Mediterranean cuisines have influenced each other for thousands of years. The origins of the domestication and cultivation of the olive tree are in Asia – the Near East, rather than in Europe. Garlic, now considered by many to be synonymous with the cooking of France, is of course a common ingredient of Asian cooking and is thought to have been introduced to Southern Europe from Central and South Asia. Trade and conquest merged cultural habits. Alexander the Great expressed respect for the civilizations he encountered on his expansion of the Macedonian Empire to India and valued their traditions including those of their diets. Enlightened peoples throughout history have embraced foreign ideas and incorporated those concepts in their own way of life. There are many other examples of ingredients brought to the markets along the spice routes from ancient times to the period of Venetian influences, including the exploits of Marco Polo and beyond. Similarities in recipes are therefore by no means coincidental. Tzatziki, the blending of yoghurt, cucumber, oil and dill is very similar to Indian raitas, meatball keftedes can be compared to koftas and the practice of wrapping rice in leaves is a common theme in both Mediterranean and Asian cooking. This breakdown of culinary borders between Europe and Asia is sometimes called the Indo-Mediterranean Diet.

It is possible to continue to explore dishes which add signature ingredients of the Mediterranean to recipes from Asia. Convention may dictate that curries are not prepared with extra virgin olive oil, and culinary purists might object, but as we have seen, taste preference is acquired and need not be fixed forever. New ways of embracing the fusion of cuisines are long established in history. Now we are aware of the health benefits of some specific elements of the Mediterranean Diet, there is the opportunity to combine the best of all worlds.

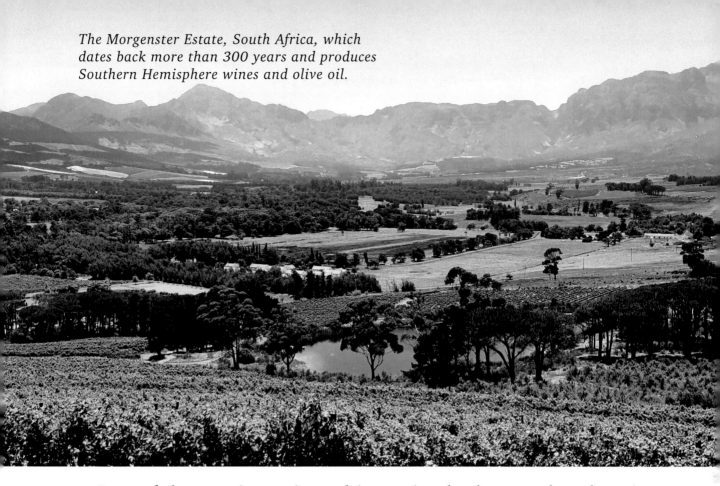

The Morgenster Estate, South Africa, which dates back more than 300 years and produces Southern Hemisphere wines and olive oil.

Some of the most innovative and interesting developments have been in "MediterrAsian" food where Mediterranean and Japanese chefs have worked together to look at novel tastes. Although this has not been promoted on the basis of health (trainee chefs often miss out on training in nutrition to a similar shocking extent as medical students) there could be an interesting academic debate on the nutritional benefits of combining miso – fermented soybeans with koji (a fungus) and extra virgin olive oil, garlic, vinegar, with tahini (the paste from crushed sesame seeds used in hummus which was possibly first brought to the Mediterranean from Ethiopia). Japan has the greatest consumption of extra virgin olive oil in Asia, and this continues to increase year on year. Most is currently imported from Spain and Italy, but there is an emerging domestic production mainly in the Mediterranean climate on the island of Shodoshima.

As we understand the importance of diet in the prevention of chronic disease and the promotion of optimum health, it is possible to take the principles and ingredients of the gold standard Mediterranean Diet and bring them to whichever diet is most familiar to us in whichever part of the world we inhabit. It is possible to "Mediterraneanise" our diets and use sustainable local produce as well as those "signature" foods of the Mediterranean which have been imported or are now grown on all of continents with a history of human habitation.

The Mediterranean Diet must be supported through education and advocacy in the face of the rise of convenience and ultra-processed foods. As we understand the subtleties of its effects, we learn more about this way of life which provides the gift of health to humans. We live in exciting times. Research is providing us with insights into the secrets of the diet. We are learning not only about the importance of basic nutritional laws, but also the importance of food colour, quality, preparation and synergistic effects as well as nature's ingenious ways of conceiving protective mastery over oxidation and inflammation. We are revealing the intuitive ways in which the inhabitants of the Mediterranean have developed over centuries a lifestyle which confers such triumph over chronic illness. Yet this knowledge will have no benefit if the majority of people have not heard of it. Understanding the way the diet works to confer benefits of health and longevity is key to achieving success with the Mediterranean Diet. Armed with this knowledge we may at least begin to make choices which can have a powerful impact on our destiny in an otherwise confusing world, and reverse the consequences of the environment of so-called convenience foods in which we live.

Summary

The principles of the Mediterranean Diet can be applied to ways of eating in other parts of the world.

The Mediterranean Diet shares many qualities in common with other traditional heritage diets.

We need to be alert to inaccurate representations or hijacking of the Mediterranean Diet.

Combining local ingredients with those of the Mediterranean Diet can give us the best of both worlds.

Extra virgin olive oil is a fundamental pillar of the Mediterranean Diet.

Part Two

From Understanding to Achieving Your
Mediterranean Diet in a Week

Chapter Ten

Ten Ways to Make the Mediterranean Diet Deliver

"We can make a commitment to promote vegetables and fruits and whole grains on every part of every menu. We can make portion sizes smaller and emphasize quality over quantity. And we can help create a culture - imagine this – where our kids ask for healthy options instead of resisting them."
Michelle Obama

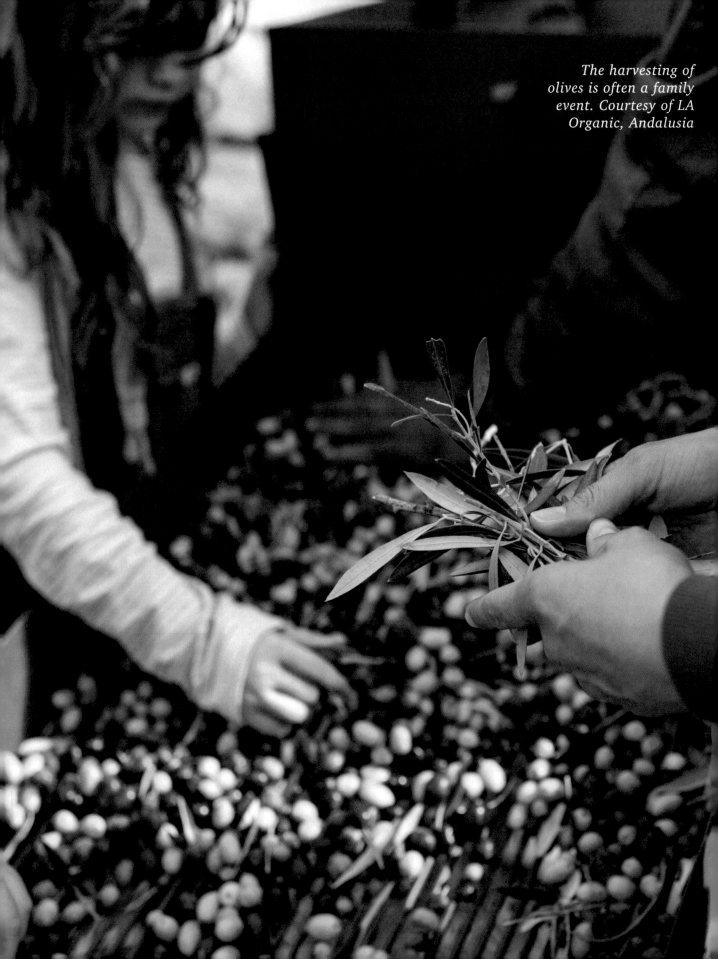

The harvesting of olives is often a family event. Courtesy of LA Organic, Andalusia

Now we know some of the secrets of the diet there are a number of ways in which we can make it really work in order to ensure it will deliver.

In order to create the benefits, we need to be aiming to achieve a low Dietary Inflammatory Index. This can be delivered through a high polyphenol Mediterranean Diet.

Here are ten simple principles to immediately adopt an effective Mediterranean Diet. We need to be familiar with the common foods described in previous chapters, understand the ways in which they work together to produce the healthiest combinations, apply the principles which are so important to the diet and finally make those simple changes to our lives to complete the transition to an excellent Mediterranean Diet.

1. Reducing our Proinflammatory Foods – Restoring Balance

Added sugars, high levels of salt and saturated fats in our diet can all have proinflammatory effects. Ultra-processed foods and those prepared or fried with high omega 6 vegetable oils also add to the Dietary Inflammatory Index. Processed meats and red meat, unless made safe in the method of cooking, may also incite inflammation.

Avoiding ingredients with chemical names which are unrecognisable is probably also a good idea, as it is to question what place they have in our foods in the first place.

Minimising or eliminating these elements in a diet at the same time as increasing anti-inflammatory foods could begin to reduce levels of chronic inflammation in a matter of days or weeks.

2. Creating a Mediterranean Shopping List

Including more vegetables, fruits, Extra Virgin Olive Oil, olives, nuts, seeds, herbs, spices, wholegrains and legumes as the plant basis of the Mediterranean Diet is a good place to start. Oily fish and poultry a few times a week. Red meat once a week or fortnight, prepared safely with Extra Virgin Olive Oil and in serving quantities consistent with a condiment to a meal of vegetables can be part of the Mediterranean Diet.

Meal and menu planning are a useful way to incorporate these ingredients into daily life. A breakfast of fruits, nuts, seeds with goat or sheep's yoghurt is an excellent way to begin the day. Salads make great lunches and olives are perfect snacks. Main meals comprised of vegetables perhaps with fish or poultry can include all the various foods of the Mediterranean Diet.

The foods are "real foods" - ingredients for meals. Foods in the traditional diet were locally sourced, so provenance and traceability was assured. Produce was organically grown not least because modern pesticides were not available.

3. Bringing Colours to the Kitchen

Polyphenols which have antioxidant properties are frequently concentrated in the colourful outer protective layers of fruits and vegetables.

Roasted, fried or raw Mediterranean vegetables are usually a rainbow of colours. Cuisine is typically vibrant and multicoloured.

In the reds, yellows, purples, blues, greens and oranges are groups of bioactive compounds with names such as flavonoids including anthocyanins and procyanidins, luteins and other carotenoids. Many of these compounds are polyphenols or related compounds with antioxidant capacity.

4. Focusing on Food quality

For those of us who might have grown our own vegetables or been at the harbour when freshly caught fish are unloaded from boats, it will be obvious that it is possible to see, smell and taste the difference between foods which are fresh and well nurtured from those which are intensively produced or not quite as fresh as we might like.

The Mediterranean Diet is based on principles of food quality. Traditional methods of farming would have preserved soil quality and supplied local markets with fresh, seasonal produce. The fruit would be grown outdoors in direct sunlight rather than in glasshouses which reduces the penetration of the UV light which can stimulate antioxidant production. The use of irrigation would be sparing as water was a precious resource, in contrast with modern intensive use of sprinklers. Crop yield is less in a more challenging and natural environment but levels of polyphenols and other antioxidants which are beneficial for health are much increased. Cheeses would, by definition be artisanal and the animals would often be roaming free to forage on a diverse intake of plants.

This is reflected in plant vitamin, mineral and polyphenols levels and also in the types and quantities of fat and proteins in animal products.

Food quality depends on the way it is produced and is reflected in taste and healthfulness.

5. Making Recipes Follow Ingredients

It is fun to select a recipe and to experiment with new ways of preparing food. The everyday Mediterranean Diet does not however need to be based on prescriptive or exact quantities or rules of cooking. It does not need to be exotic. In fact, it is often exactly the opposite. It is based on the combination of simple ingredients.

Roasting sweet potato, carrots, and parsnips with garlic in Extra Virgin Olive Oil or gently frying peppers, onions and aubergines with paprika does not have to follow a specific recipe. The ingredients themselves do not necessarily need to be from the Mediterranean. Atlantic Salmon fillets can be baked with a sprinkle of fennel seeds or parsley and a drizzle of Extra Virgin Olive Oil. A bean stew with basil and oregano in a sofrito sauce is a beautiful winter meal, and in the summer endless combinations of salads with nuts, cheeses or fruit can be finished with infused Extra Virgin Olive Oils. Chicken breasts or a small amount of red meat can be marinated in oil, wine, garlic and chilli and served with lentils or couscous cooked in chopped tomatoes with spices.

These are not recipes but combinations of common kitchen staples. All are healthy and emblematic of the Mediterranean Diet. They require the right ingredients to be present but do not need complex preparation, advanced planning or precise measurement.

6. Acquiring the Taste

Many plant compounds that are good for health are associated with interesting tastes. Carotenoids and polyphenols may give pleasant bitterness, pungency or even sourness. Garlic is rich in sulphur-based chemicals which contribute to its unique flavour and there are suggestions that it reduces the tendency to form blood clots.

Herbs and spices are common in the Mediterranean Diet and not only provide added interest and flavour to food but also are a very highly concentrated source of bioactive compounds which may have very diverse effects. These may be anti-inflammatory, antibacterial, antioxidant, analgesic (pain killing), or contribute to the health of blood vessels and reduce blood clots.

For example, the most commonly used spice in many countries is pepper. It not only has antioxidant properties but is also a "bioenhancer", increasing the absorption of selenium, vitamin B12, curcumin and beta carotene which are antioxidants in their own right.

Oregano, peppermint, cinnamon and rosemary frequently top the list of total antioxidant measurements in laboratory studies, but levels can vary as with any natural product. The antioxidant concentration per gram is much higher than fruit and vegetables though we of course consume smaller quantities of spices overall. Dried as well as fresh herbs and spices are a great source of flavour and health benefits.

7. Considering Food, from Farm to Kitchen

It is worth considering what we mean by the processing of food as it journeys from an original source to our homes. An easy short hand definition of a "processed" food might be one which contains multiple unrecognisable ingredients, and an "ultra-processed" food might feel even further removed from its natural state.

Sugars, salt, saturated fat, vegetable oils including palm oil, additives and preservatives in processed foods can have a pro-inflammatory effect contributing to chronic inflammation and therefore disease. Although we can identify what we commonly call processed foods by the list of such ingredients, strictly speaking food processing has a broader definition. Whilst foods can so often be altered to include dubious ingredients or undergo processes which lose beneficial nutrients, occasionally processing can enhance the value of a food.

For example, wine production could be defined as the processing of grapes to produce the final alcoholic beverage. Techniques of wine making vary. For example, a longer maceration time can result in higher levels of polyphenols in red wine. This is the part of wine production where the grapes are soaked, bringing out the flavours and colours of the polyphenols of the skin and raising the levels of polyphenols including tannins, catechins and proanthocyanidins thought to confer health benefits.

Strictly speaking Extra Virgin Olive Oil is a processed food, by virtue of the olives undergoing a mechanical pressing to extract the oil. Of course, this creates a very healthy and natural product - the "freshly squeezed fruit juice" of the olive.

On the other hand, when olives have their stones removed an additional washing process is applied which removes a substantial quantity of the polyphenols.

Table olives are themselves a product of processing, and whilst this changes some of the polyphenol content, rather special healthy nutrients remain. The Romans discovered that olives, usually palatable only to birds, could have much of the bitterness removed by placing them in brine and sodium hydroxide found in wood ash, rather than the previous lengthy and laborious methods of repeatedly soaking and washing the olive with salt water. There is a rather engageing story told of the first discovery of this processing method. It was said that a young Roman child was found at harvest time amidst the ash of a long-abandoned fire where peasants had been cooking their lunch. He was picking up the fallen olives and enjoying their taste because they had been naturally "processed" from lying in the burnt wood. Although table olives are considered a very healthy part of the Mediterranean Diet, their packageing in brine can add unwanted salt to the diet or presentation in sunflower oil increase unnecessarily our already high levels of omega 6 fats from vegetable and seed oils. Riper olives can be naturally deep purple or brown in colour but are distinct from black table olives first produced in California. These are not olives which have ripened from green to black on the tree. They have undergone a technique of curing in an alkaline solution and treated with oxygen and iron. They have little bitterness as a result of the loss of much of their polyphenol content.

Similarly, the skins of nuts are particularly rich in polyphenols in their outer layers. A handful of raw nuts is a common snack in the Mediterranean. In many countries however nuts are processed to remove the skins as well as being salted and roasted. This diminishes their nutritional value.

Honey is valued in the Mediterranean, where it is traditionally eaten in its original, natural state. Many consumers are unaware that much of the commercially-produced honey undergoes processing involving pasteurisation and fine filtering. This is done predominantly for cosmetic and convenience reasons, to maintain the honey in liquid form for longer on the shelf. Although honey is rich in sugars there is no evidence that consumption in moderation increases the risk of obesity or diabetes. Apart from the sugars, unprocessed honey is a rich source of antioxidant, anti-inflammatory and antibacterial micronutrients produced by the bees for protection from environmental threats. These elements may be reduced by the heating during pasteurisation. It is often difficult to discern honeys which are processed from those which are in their original form. Some producers of artisan honey are beginning to communicate the advantages of their methods of production to consumers and describing it as "raw honey".

There are many other stories of processing which alters the nutritional value of foods, occasionally for good, but more often with a detrimental effect.

It is always advisable to look at the label and to ask questions about how food is processed and produced and what effects that may have on its final quality.

8. Considering Food, from Kitchen to Table

Food preparation techniques commonly used in the Mediterranean region influence how nutrients are preserved and made most available for absorption.

Foods are in general cooked together. Boiling, or to a lesser extent, steaming results in the loss of nutrients to the cooking water. In contrast, marinating and cooking in Extra Virgin Olive Oil allows for the beneficial transfer, greater availability and increased absorption of bioactive antioxidant and anti-inflammatory polyphenols, vitamin D and other micronutrients. It also reduces the production and absorption of potentially harmful compounds which might otherwise be a product of cooking processes, protects and secures more fragile and heat sensitive nutrients and enhances the diversity of the beneficial gastrointestinal microbiome.

Moreover, the kitchen is a place of energy and of communal activity. It is the sacred heart of a Mediterranean home. Eating for pleasure is a pillar of the Mediterranean Diet. Portion sizes are modest and meals are usually enjoyed slowly and in company. There is evidence to suggest that this is more likely to reduce overall calorie intake and to ensure early satiety. The importance of sharing meals as a social experience is key to a greater focus on food quality and a value placed on taste even for the simplest of meals. The traditional Mediterranean Diet is based on an intuitive food consciousness and literacy which is passed down from generation to generation. Enjoying food together has a status of great social importance and meaning.

9. Understanding the Central Role of Quality Extra Virgin Olive Oil

Good quality Extra Virgin Olive Oil is at the heart of the Mediterranean diet. It is used for preparation, cooking and the finishing of dishes. It is a part of every meal and is present in significant quantity. It has independent, measurable and significant health benefits as an anti-inflammatory and antioxidant food as well as regulating glycaemic effects. It is the cornerstone of the diet and at least two or three tablespoons per person per day are commonly used.

In particular the high polyphenol oils which are identifiable for their harmony of fruitiness, bitterness and pungency have powerful properties.

10. Drinking for Health

When it comes to keeping healthily hydrated, there is by definition no substitute for water.

Sodas and carbonated drinks often contain significant amounts of salt and sugar, or contain replacement artificial sweeteners. A good place to start is to eliminate soda drinks and to enjoy the simple refreshment of water, perhaps with a slice of lemon.

Drinking wine, especially red wine, in moderation and with an extra virgin oil rich meal can be an enjoyable part of the Mediterranean Diet. Wine polyphenols have the potential to contribute to heart health.

Teas are commonly consumed as part of the Mediterranean Diet. Herbal teas as well as green or black teas can be rich sources of antioxidants. Particular teas are unique to regions of the Mediterranean including, for example the wild gathered sereritis "mountain tea" of Greece which is attracting the attention of academics interested in researching health properties of specific traditional drinks.

Summary

Achieve a basic Mediterranean Diet with an unprocessed, real food, plant predominant diet.

Graduate to excellence with a polyphenol rich diet based on quality and colour.

Expand taste experience with the flavours of health bestowing bioactive compounds.

Supercharge the Mediterranean Diet food combinations with Extra Virgin Olive Oil.

Enjoy alcohol the Mediterranean way.

Chapter Eleven

How Mediterranean is Your Diet?
Take the 20 Question Quiz

"The secret of change is to focus all your energy not on
fighting the old, but on building the new."
Socrates

At the beginning of the plan described in the next chapter, take the quiz and calculate your score. This will give you a rough idea how Mediterranean your current diet is (adding one question on exercise to reflect an active lifestyle), and provide a challenge to increase your score over the week. It is important to note that the scores are not weighted for relative importance so should be used only as a general guide. For those who are vegetarian or abstain from alcohol, total scores can be adjusted to reflect a vegetarian or alcohol free Mediterranean Diet and the relevant questions ignored.

	Question	Scores 1	Scores 0	Total
1	How many servings of vegetables do you eat each day? (1 serving = approx. 100g includes medium salads which may weigh less than 100g)	5 or More	4 or Fewer	
2	How many different colours of vegetables do you eat in each main meal?	3 or More	2 or Fewer	
3	How many servings of fruit do you eat each day? (1 serving = approx. 100g)	3 or More	2 or Fewer	
4	How many times a week do you consume different legumes or pulses such as lentils, chickpeas, peas and beans?	3 or More	2 or Fewer	
5	How many times a week do you consume wholegrains?	3 or More	2 or Fewer	
6	Do you use extra virgin olive oil for all types of cooking and as your only oil?	Yes	No	
7	How much good quality (regionally identifiable – see guide to buying) extra virgin olive oil do you consume each day?	3 or More Tablespoons	2 or Fewer Tablespoons	
8	Do you regularly eat seafood cooked (oven or pan) with extra virgin olive oil?	Yes	No	
9	How many times a week do you eat a handful (approx. 30g) of unsalted, raw nuts (excluding peanuts)?	5 or More	4 or Fewer	
10	How many times a week do you eat sweets, commercial bakery products e.g. pastries, ice cream?	2 or Fewer	3 or More	

11	Do you consume no red meat, or occasionally, always prepared with extra virgin olive oil, in maximum portion size 120g, maximum frequency once per week?	Yes	No	
12	Do you eat processed meat for example sausages and bacon and processed convenience foods less than once per week?	Yes	No	
13	Do you eat unsweetened yoghurt and unprocessed cheese as your main intake of dairy rather than butter, cream and margarine?	Yes	No	
14	Do you eat "scratch" main meals i.e. home prepared using fresh ingredients more than 5 times per week.	Yes	No	
15	How many days a week do you add a variety of herbs and spices to cooking?	5 or More	4 or Fewer	
16	How many times do you prepare a sauce similar to sofrito each week? (olive oil, garlic, onions, tomatoes)	2 or More	1 or Fewer	
17	Do you consume two or more of the following regularly each week – high cocoa chocolate, raw honey or olives?	Yes	No	
18	Do you regularly (weekly) drink products with added sugars or sugar substitutes for examples pops and sodas?	No	Yes	
19	If you consume alcohol is it always wine, in moderation (less than 250mls per day) with a meal rich in extra virgin olive oil	Yes	No	
20	Do you get at least 150 minutes of moderate aerobic activity or 75 minutes of vigorous aerobic activity a week, or a combination of moderate and vigorous activity?	Yes	No	

Results

Score 15 – 20
You are doing really well. Keep up the good work. See what small additional changes you can make to perfect your Mediterranean Diet.

Score 10-15
You are on the right track. There is room for improvement to make real gains. Focus on a few of the areas to improve your score

Score 5-10
There is lots of work you can do. Concentrate on your vegetables and extra virgin olive oil to get some easy wins and work from there

Score 0-5
The good news is that there is so much you can do to improve your diet. Using the menus and the tips from this book, you can at least double your score in a matter of days!

Chapter Twelve

An Introduction to the 7-Day Mediterranean Diet Programme

"One day the trees went out to anoint a king for themselves. They said to the olive tree, 'Be our king.' But the olive tree answered, 'Should I give up my oil, by which both gods and humans are honored, to hold sway over the trees?'
The Old Testament, Judges 9

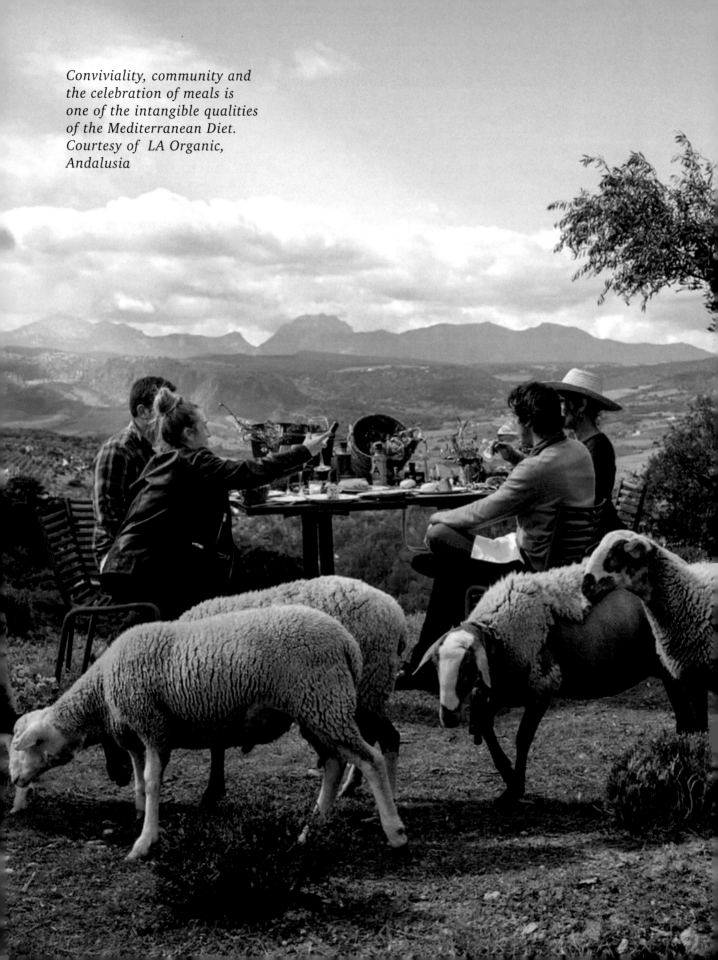

*Conviviality, community and
the celebration of meals is
one of the intangible qualities
of the Mediterranean Diet.
Courtesy of LA Organic,
Andalusia*

Following this 7-day programme will help you to get started on your more Mediterranean Diet. The plan can be used as a guide and need not be followed strictly. The menus for the 7 days are a practical illustration of the principles of moving to a more Mediterranean Diet to feel happier and healthier. This is a journey which involves:

- Removing processed foods and always reading food labels. Avoiding the unrecognisable.

- Shopping for the "real food" staples of the Mediterranean Diet with meal combination planning

- Focusing on anti-inflammatory polyphenol rich colourful vegetables at the heart of meals

- Learning to recognise quality in foods from ancient grains and "slow" foods nurtured carefully to well-reared meat and dairy

- Stocking up on great ingredients to have to hand – from lemon juice and vinegars to nuts, seeds and other healthy condiments

- Experimenting with the tastes of herbs and spices.

- Enjoying good quality extra virgin olive oil – at least 2 tablespoons per day for health, flavour and pleasure

- Cooking with ingredient combinations, always with extra virgin olive oil and including the cooking juices with the meal– creating the magic alchemy of the Mediterranean Diet

- For those who choose to drink alcohol, consuming mainly wine, in moderation and always with a Mediterranean extra virgin olive oil rich meal.

There is some research suggesting that sugar and salt intake can be gradually reduced and taste preferences will adapt. There is debate about whether cravings from sugar and salt represent an "addiction" in the true sense of the word, but what is clear is that a steady decrease in the amounts consumed will result in a greater sensitivity to the taste. In other words, weaning off salt and sugar means they are not missed. Adding ingredients such as herbs and spices and extra virgin olive oil will increase the variety of flavours including spicy, peppery and pleasant bitter tones to foods.

A Plan for Every Day

The plan includes meals where simplicity is the key. Recipes with specific instructions may take a little longer to prepare and can be reserved for days when there is more time available to spend in the kitchen. This follows research which shows that for most people it is easier to achieve and sustain a healthy diet by cooking from scratch using straightforward combinations of ingredients most days of the week. The Mediterranean Diet is learned through knowledge of its elements, principles and patterns rather than having to refer to a cookbook each night of a busy week. Lunch suggestions in the plan are convenient for eating at home, taking to work or school. The pattern of eating is perfect for children as well as older people. Frozen vegetables may replace fresh vegetables and dried herbs may be substituted for fresh herbs when appropriate. Tinned products are sometimes as good as fresh foods but ensure the ingredients do not include added preservatives or sugars.

It is common practice in the Mediterranean to eat food left over from one day in a subsequent meal or snack. Food waste is kept to a minimum which is beneficial for the environment and also for the budget. If there is a little too much rice it can be conveniently and tastily added to a cold salad for lunch the following day. Vegetables not consumed in a meal can be added to a stew on another occasion.

When it comes to drinks, many people have become used to sugary carbonated brands. Longer lasting refreshment with taste comes with adding freshly squeezed citrus fruits such as lemons, limes or oranges including perhaps segments of the fruit to water. Lemon juice has also been shown to reduce the glycaemic load of a meal, helping to reduce spikes in blood sugar levels.

A Healthy Weight Loss Programme – The End of Dieting

Many books make astonishing claims about rapid weight loss on a plan which might focus on eradicating a particular macronutrient, include a dramatic reduction in calories or a combination of both, without heed to any potential harm to other aspects of health. A diet where healthy fats are replaced with poor quality carbohydrates, or conversely where the benefits of wholegrain carbohydrates are lost and substituted with red meat may result in weight reduction but the nutritional risks are clear. Evidence is accumulating that any weight loss from such diets is generally short lived and these kinds of eating patterns are unlikely to be sustainable or healthy in the long term.

In contrast, the Mediterranean Diet is a way of life which involves modest portion sizes, the right types, quality and proportion of macronutrients and a culture of eating slowly and consciously. It is a pattern of eating which beats other diets for sustained and manageable reduction in weight from an overweight to normal range. It is protective against obesity for several reasons – the predominance of extra virgin olive oil as the main source of fat, the low GI carbohydrates, the sense of fullness gained from plant proteins high in fibre, as well as the contribution from micronutrients and bioactive compounds such as polyphenols which are capable of beneficial effects on hormones and genes which influence metabolism. The way foods are combined together also has an effect on the absorption and handling of the sugars consumed in a meal. At the same time, the diet reduces the risk of type 2 diabetes and lowers blood pressure. It delivers reductions in risk of many other chronic conditions including heart disease, stroke, many types of cancers and diseases related to obesity and chronic inflammation.

Adopting a Mediterranean Diet may result in an immediate decrease in markers of chronic inflammation for those who seek a reduction in weight as well as people who may be a healthy weight to begin with. Although this is not something which can be shown by jumping on the bathroom scales, these effects are even more important than losing weight quickly. In order to lose weight with a Mediterranean Diet it is important to set a target in terms of how much and how quickly. A change from a standard western diet to a Mediterranean lifestyle will provide a path from an obesogenic diet to one which is associated with a healthy BMI – the Body Mass Index number which combines figures of height and weight to determine if an individual is in a category of underweight, normal, overweight or obese. The speed at which this can be achieved depends on how closely the diet is adhered to and how significant is the reduction in portion size. Simply counting calories is less useful since the calorific values for foods do not very accurately predict their effect on weight.

Whilst a useful guide, Body Mass Index does have limitations since a person's weight may reflect muscle rather than fat, and it may be a less useful measurement of health in older people. A Mediterranean Diet has been shown to be protective for people in the overweight range, reducing the increased risks associated with increasing BMI. The mortality rate over twenty years in people of normal BMI with a low adherence to the Mediterranean Diet was actually higher than that of people who adhered to a Mediterranean Diet and who were classified as overweight.

Following this programme will take you to a more Mediterranean Diet in 7 days. This is a diet which research has shown to be associated not only with reduced rates of chronic disease and with a healthy weight but also a sense of wellbeing, improved mood, enhanced exercise performance and fitness. This might well be described as an opportunity for delivering a leaner, fitter, healthier and happier you. The credibility is not in the promises of a celebrity with an impossibly "perfect" waistline or a nutritionist selling an implausible new formula of shakes. The authority of the diet is in the published science. The integrity and the validity are in the evidence.

The Mediterranean Diet for Omnivores and for Vegetarians

The Mediterranean Diet is a plant-based diet. The majority of foods are vegetables and legumes, with fish and meat added in relatively smaller quantities. A meat predominant meal would be traditionally served on feast days, perhaps once a month. For the translation of the Mediterranean Diet to the present day and western cultures, a reasonable reinterpretation of this might be to eat red meat once a week or fortnight, but with palm sized portions of good quality meat prepared safely with an extra virgin olive oil and vegetable rich meal. All the meals described in this programme can be modified to be vegetarian with little effort or explanation. Protein replacement for meat can be achieved with pulses such as beans, lentils and peas or nuts, tofu and other soy-based products or mycoprotein. Cheeses such as halloumi can also be incorporated.

It has Got to Be Extra Virgin Olive Oil in the Kitchen

Extra virgin olive oil is fundamental to the Mediterranean Diet. It is the only oil used for cooking in the traditional Mediterranean Diet and is the only oil included in the 7-day plan.

The antioxidant content of extra virgin olive oil is uniquely high and is far greater than that of other oils.

Antioxidants protect the fruit of the olive tree from the damageing effects of oxidation in the environment.

Antioxidants also protect human cells from oxidative stress which can result in chronic inflammatory processes, cell ageing and damage, cancers, heart disease, stroke, dementia and many other diseases of chronic inflammation.

Antioxidants protect an oil from the effects of heat. High temperatures during cooking accelerate chemical reactions including oxidative breakdown of the oil, resulting in the breakdown of fats to release free fatty acids and formation of potentially harmful chemicals many of which can behave as free radicals. So called "polar compounds" are formed from the oxidation of the fats. The total polar compound level is a reliable benchmark for the measurement of degradation of an oil. Many of these polar compounds have been associated with increased risks of cancers and Alzheimer's disease.

The antioxidants in extra virgin olive oil protect it from oxidation during cooking, and so reduce the formation of polar compounds and free radicals. Some of these antioxidants will be sacrificed in the protection and preservation of the oil, but at usual cooking temperatures, as much as 40% of the original antioxidant capacity remains (depending on temperature and the length of the heat exposure). Higher levels of antioxidants in an oil and lower levels of polar compounds formed after heating indicate the healthiest oils to use for cooking. In the case of an extra virgin olive oil with a good level of polyphenol antioxidants in the first place, it will be an excellent oil to use for cooking, with enough antioxidant capacity to preserve it through the cooking process and plenty left over to provide health benefits when the food is consumed, enhanced with a drizzle of fresh oil on the dish.

We also see that the antioxidants in the extra virgin olive oil protect other foods from oxidation during heating and, perhaps even more importantly, cooking results in the combination and exchange of antioxidants between foods which creates the potential to be even more healthily available to the body.

Table 1 shows levels of total antioxidants in different oils. Much of the antioxidant capacity of some of these oils may be derived from a small number of antioxidants like Vitamin E. It should be noted however that the power of antioxidants for human health may well depend on the synergistic effects of different antioxidants. A further advantage of extra virgin olive oil therefore is in the numerous varieties of polyphenols which act in addition to the antioxidant effect of Vitamin E.

Table 2 shows the levels of potentially harmful polar compounds formed when oils are subjected to heating. These results represent average levels following heating at temperatures between 25 and 240 degrees centigrade from 30 to 360 minutes. Extra virgin olive oil demonstrates the lowest formation of polar compounds across high temperatures and for prolonged periods.

Table 1

Oil Type	Antioxidant Content in mg/kg
Extra Virgin Olive Oil	5972
Virgin Olive Oil	4949
Olive Oil	3281
Avocado	936
Canola	327
Peanut	283
Sunflower	275
Coconut	8

Table 2

Oil Type	Final Polar Compounds Percentage in Oil
Extra Virgin Olive Oil	8.47
Virgin Olive Oil	10.71
Olive Oil	11.65
Grapeseed Oil	19.79
Avocado Oil	11.60
Coconut Oil	9.30
Sunflower Oil	15.57
Rice Bran Oil	14.35
Peanut Oil	10.71

Reproduced by kind permission of Dr Claudia Guillaume. First Published in Acta Scientific Nutritional Health, *Volume 2, Issue 6. (June 2018)*

Chapter Thirteen

Preparing for The Seven Day Programme

"Give me six hours to chop down a tree and I will spend
the first four sharpening the axe."
Abraham Lincoln

We begin with a focus on bringing home the foods that will be the foundation of our Mediterranean Diet. Some of these foods can be bought at a supermarket or local convenience store. Others are best found in health food shops or even bought online, where bulk purchases may be more economic. Farmers' markets are increasingly popular and are often a source of good quality fresh local produce. This replicates the way in which most shopping is done in more traditional areas of the Mediterranean, where growers bring fruit and vegetables to nearby towns and villages.

Before making a list of ingredients to buy, see what staples are already in the cupboards and the freezer. It may not be affordable or practical to buy all these foods on the first shop, so consider making a rolling list to build up week by week. To continue beyond the first week, it is good to have the following foods with long shelf life readily available:

For the Cupboards
- Extra Virgin Olive Oil
- Wholegrain rice
- Couscous
- Quinoa
- Lentils
- Oats
- Whole-wheat, spelt or other types of pasta
- Flour – spelt and other ancient varieties
- Beans and Chickpeas – dried, or tinned (without added preservatives)
- Passata or Tinned Tomatoes
- Raw Honey
- Dried Herbs
- Vinegars including Balsamic Vinegar
- Pomegranate molasses
- Tahini
- Dark Chocolate minimum 70% cocoa
- Dried fruits such as dates, raisins etc
- Nuts and Seeds
- Olives
- Varieties of Teas
- Full Bodied Ground Coffee

For the Freezer
- Frozen Vegetables
- Frozen Beans
- Prepacked Frozen Herbs, Chilli, Garlic, Ginger where available (chillies can be frozen from fresh)
- Frozen Fruits including berries

For the Fridge or Stored in a Cool Place
- Fresh Vegetables
- Salad Ingredients
- Fresh Fruit
- Yoghurt
- Cheeses
- Eggs
- Quality Bread
- Fresh herbs

Add to the list the portions of fish, poultry or other meat which are going to compliment your week's plant-based Mediterranean Diet. It is best to choose these guided by the recommendations of the butcher or fishmonger and to buy fresh and seasonal cuts or fillets. All the menus for the week can substitute different fish or meat. It is a tradition of the Mediterranean region to have high expectations and to closely examine and smell what is on offer. You will be amazed at how such interactions can become an engageing and enjoyable part of the shopping experience. If there is insufficient time to always buy fresh fish or meat, freezing is a possibility for added convenience.

Aim for a kitchen which mirrors the Mediterranean Diet Pyramid illustrated previously.

Phase out any stocks of unhealthy convenience or processed foods and ensure that every food in your kitchen has ingredients which are recognisable and natural.

Having prepared the kitchen, now is the time to begin the 7-day programme to achieve and sustain a more Mediterranean Diet.

Chapter Fourteen

A Seven Day Menu Planner

"Everything should be made as simple as possible, but
not simpler."
Albert Einstein

EVOO = Extra Virgin Olive Oil

	Breakfast	**Lunch**	**Dinner**
Day 1	Porridge with a teaspoon of raw honey, a dash of cinnamon and a drizzle of extra virgin olive oil	Salad leaves with tomatoes, chopped fennel, orange slices, pomegranate seeds, and walnuts. Slice of ancient seed bread and EVOO	Oily fish (tuna, salmon, sea bass, trout) fillet baked with EVOO and herbs served with wholegrain rice and fresh chopped spring onions. Green vegetable to accompany – EVOO sautéed greens or courgettes with ginger and cumin seeds. Rice may be finished off fried with vegetables
Day 2	Fresh fruit with nuts, seeds and Greek yoghurt. Fresh mint leaves if available	Rice salad (prepared Day 1 dinner) with combinations of sun-dried tomatoes, peas, sweet corn, chopped yellow and red peppers, pine nuts, feta cheese, fresh basil and onions with an EVOO dressing	Vegetarian bean stew – soak beans overnight or cook from frozen/ tinned. Slow cook/ oven casserole mixed beans with plenty of EVOO, passata or tinned tomatoes and vegetable stock. Add frozen or fresh vegetables or broccoli, black pepper, turmeric, chopped chillies, garlic and red onions.

	Breakfast	**Lunch**	**Dinner**
Day 3	Herb sprinkled extra virgin olive oil fried eggs on sourdough/ ancient grain bread	Chickpea salad with combinations of avocado, cubed pecorino, manchego or other hard cheese, chopped cucumber, onions, tomatoes, olives, lemon juice or balsamic vinegar with extra virgin olive oil. Parsley to garnish	Roasted Chicken breasts in EVOO and Cajun mixed spices or paprika. 10 minutes before serving can be stuffed with mozzarella and/ or wrapped in Parma ham. At the same time roast in EVOO accompanying mixed vegetables – finely sliced sweet potato, aubergines (eggplants) and leeks or bell peppers.
Day 4	Granola (low sugar) with skimmed milk or kefir.	Couscous or quinoa (prepared the night before) salad with diced tomatoes, cucumber, pickled beetroot, raisins or dried apricots with honey and Dijon mustard EVOO dressing.	Seafood and pea pasta bake. Defrost or prepare fresh seafood- prawns, scallops, squid, mussels and EVOO fry with chillies, ginger or saffron, garlic and spring onions and add passata. Meanwhile prepare the pasta al dente and steam the peas. Add together and finish off in the oven with a mozzarella topping.

	Breakfast	**Lunch**	**Dinner**
Day 5	Berries (fresh blueberries and strawberries or defrosted berries) and nuts and seeds with goat or sheep yoghurt and a shower of nutmeg	Pasta, tuna and bean salad. Cold pasta cooked Day 4 combined with tuna in extra virgin olive oil, beans and an EVOO dressing	Field mushrooms baked in EVOO adorned with halloumi cheese, finished under the grill and curried lentils. Boil the lentils for a few minutes until soft and then add to the frying pan with sautéed red onions, garlic and passata. Curry paste or curry spices to taste.
Day 6	Sofrito – extra virgin olive oil fried onions, garlic, tomatoes on rye bread or toast	Rye bread with various toppings of anchovies, sardines, guacamole or hummus (pureed chickpeas, tahini, garlic, lemon juice, EVOO) with salad leaf garnish	White fish (hake, halibut, cod etc) or oily fish baked in EVOO with rosemary and oregano (fresh or dried) butternut squash boiled and then mashed with EVOO and combined with sautéed garlic and onion. Serve with minted peas.
Day 7	Omelette with extra virgin olive oil fried onions, mushrooms, peppers and herbs	Soup. A good investment is a soup making machine – follow the instructions to prepare many combinations of vegetable soups with herbs and spices to taste.	Small portion of good quality beef steak, lamb fillet or Iberian presa with mixed, colourful EVOO roasted root vegetables – potatoes, parsnips and carrots with French beans.

The menu is constructed with slightly more preparation required for meals on day 6 and 7, assuming those to be days with a little more time. Lunches on days 1 to 5 can be prepared the evening before or prepared in less than 5 minutes on the day and taken to work, school or eaten at home.

All the dishes on the menu are improved with a drizzle of extra virgin olive oil. Store some at work or in small transportable bottles for travelling.

Desserts are generally suggested to be pieces of fruit. This can be made special with a little balsamic vinegar drizzled on top, or at a weekend perhaps baked in EVOO and honey with cinnamon and raisins, served with yoghurt and walnut pieces or seeds. Cheese, dates or a small amount of dark chocolate can also provide a taste contrast with fruit at the end of a meal.

Snacks during the day are perfectly acceptable – olives, raw unsalted nuts or pieces of fruit, fresh or dried.

Ingredients are key to achieving the best Mediterranean Diet. The 7-day programme provides a template for continuing to apply the principles of the diet for life by mixing up the style of dishes day by day. Look upon the foods of the Mediterranean Diet as the keys on a piano – by exploring different combinations there are so many meal compositions we can create.

For special occasions there is the possibility of following specific recipes to achieve the harmony of tastes inspired by the amazing talents of leading chefs.

Part Three

Recipes from Leading Chefs of the
Mediterranean Diet

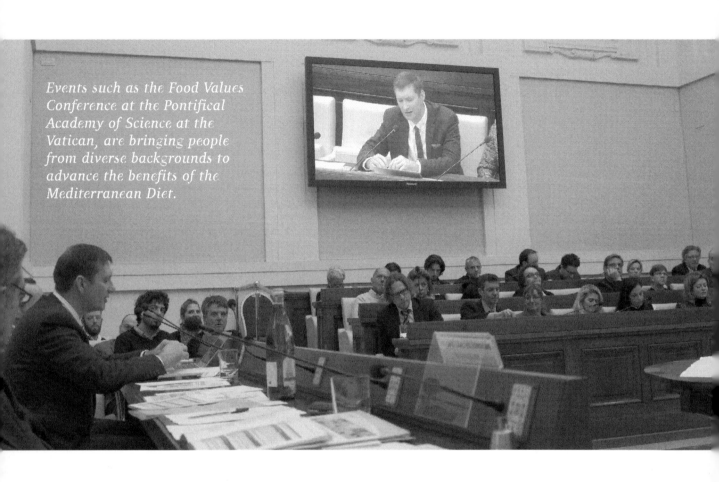

Events such as the Food Values Conference at the Pontifical Academy of Science at the Vatican, are bringing people from diverse backgrounds to advance the benefits of the Mediterranean Diet.

It has been a privilege to meet many extraordinary people who work to promote the Mediterranean Diet. There are epidemiologists influencing public policy, scientists at the cutting edge of research, health professionals passionately advocating lifestyle changes to their patients, farmers working tirelessly to perfect the quality of their produce and writers who inspire new audiences to adopt the diet.

When enthusiasts of the Mediterranean Diet from diverse backgrounds come together in forums to debate and discuss this ancient way of life there are always new lessons to be learned. The conclusions invariably return to the importance of sharing stories, understanding the diet, improving education and encourageing and enabling people to adopt it for the sake of their health and a sustainable planet.

Chefs, like doctors, have the potential to be great influencers and yet in the past received little training in nutrition. We are fortunate however to have many who inspire us through their knowledge of the Mediterranean way of life and who demonstrate this in their work – chefs who educate, preserve the traditions and are also at the vanguard of new concepts in the evolving story of the Mediterranean Diet.

This section includes some favourite recipes from these ambassadors of healthy Mediterranean cuisine. They show the breadth and scope of the extraordinary work they do. Some have chosen simple recipes which can be prepared at home, others have shared the secrets of the inventive creations which can be experienced in their restaurants. I am deeply indebted to those who have contributed and am privileged to count as friends these internationally celebrated and highly influential chefs who practice their culinary art and express their interpretation of the Mediterranean Diet in every part of the world. It is possible to travel from one country to another and see great chefs bringing traditional recipes from a grandparent's kitchen to New York, London or Paris, or returning home from Madrid, Naples or Tunis with a passion for the aromas and tastes of the city's markets and restaurants.

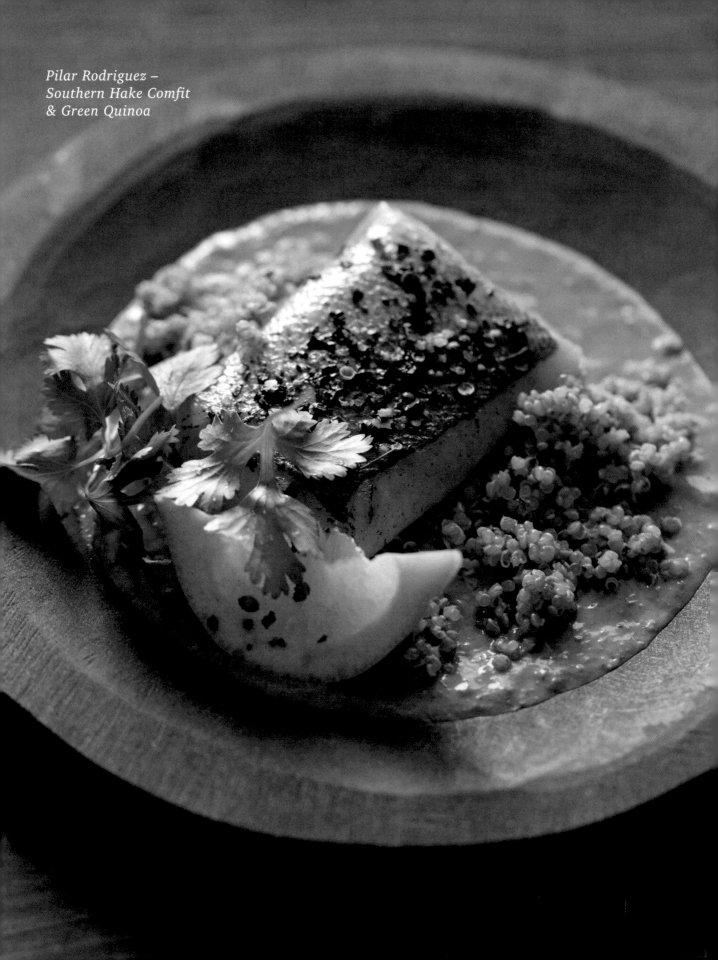

Pilar Rodriguez –
Southern Hake Comfit
& Green Quinoa

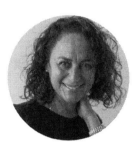

Pilar Rodriguez
Chile

Chilean celebrity chef Pilar Rodriguez is renowned for her work with Chilean Extra Virgin Olive Oil and wines and for culinary expressions of the Mediterranean Diet using local South American produce. She runs the Food & Wine Studio based in Chile's Colchagua Valley, 130km southeast of the country's capital, Santiago. A frequent star of TV, magazine and other media work she is an exemplar of New World cuisine for health as well as taste.

Southern Hake Comfit
& Green Quinoa

Serves: 1

Complexity:

Ingredients

1/4 cup Extra Virgin Olive Oil
4 southern hake fillets 150 grams each
400 mls of Extra Virgin Olive Oil for confit (usually I use leccino variety)
2 bay leaves
10 black peppercorns
3 garlic cloves

Hake rub
20 grams of merkén
20 grams of fleur de sel
20 grams of ground coriander seeds

Green Quinoa
2 cups of cooked quinoa
100 grams of whole fresh parsley
2 or 3 green onion (only the green part)
10 mint leaves
150 mls of Extra Virgin Olive Oil
Sea salt and pepper to taste
Juice of half a fresh lemon
1 avocado (hass type)

Method

1. For the Green Quinoa: Process the parsley, chives (the green part), mint, lemon juice and Extra Virgin Olive Oil until they form a paste. Flavor with salt and pepper as desired. Add to the cooked quinoa. Pass it through a strainer and separate the

pulp and the sauce. Add the pulp to the cooked quinoa and seasoned with salt and pepper. Reserve the sauce. Purée the avocado in the blender and mix with green sauce. Reserve.

2. Mix the salt with the merkén and the coriander seeds and reserve. Confit the hake fillets in Extra Virgin Olive Oil with bay leaf, garlic and pepper at 60°C for approximately 15 to 20 minutes, cook until you get a pearly white colour in the centre of the fish. It is important that the oil does not rise in temperature, otherwise it will fry the fish.

3. Once cooked, remove from the oil and dry over paper. Serve with the green quinoa and green sauce, rub the fish with the mixture of coriander seeds, merkén and sea salt. Serve immediately.

Wine Pairing

The smoky notes provided by the merkén and other mentholated coriander seeds are well received by a Moscatel de Itata, fresh and with good acidity that balances the fat of the southern hake and the avocado, refreshed, in turn, for the quinoa and herbs.

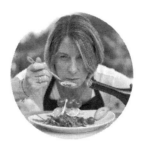

Fabienne Codaccioni Roux
France

Born in Marseille in the South of France, Fabienne is an International Olive Oil Council international expert "From Tree to Plate". She is a sommelier, educator and coach. She is an international Extra Virgin Olive Oil judge with over thirty years of experience and is the Director of Educational Programmes for the Women in Olive Oil initiative.

Pistou Soup
A Tradition of Provençal cuisine

Serves: 4-6

Complexity:

Ingredients

150g of green beans
300g of white beans
300g of red beans
300g of flat beans
1 tomato
1 zucchini (courgette)

1 potato
1 onion
2 cloves of garlic
1 sprig of fresh basil.
100g of grated parmesan cheese
Extra Virgin Olive Oil

Method

1. Prepare all the vegetables, wash and shell the beans (red and white)

2. Cut the other green vegetables into small square pieces.

3. Place all the vegetables except the potato and tomatoes into a large saucepan with water and a sprig of basil and cook for approximately 45 minutes until the red beans are tender.

4. Add the potato in small pieces and the whole tomato and simmer for approximately 15 minutes more.

5. To make the pistou- remove the tomato and crush with the garlic cloves, basil leaves and Extra Virgin Olive Oil and add to the soup.

6. Season and serve with grated parmesan cheese and a generous drizzle of Extra Virgin Olive Oil.

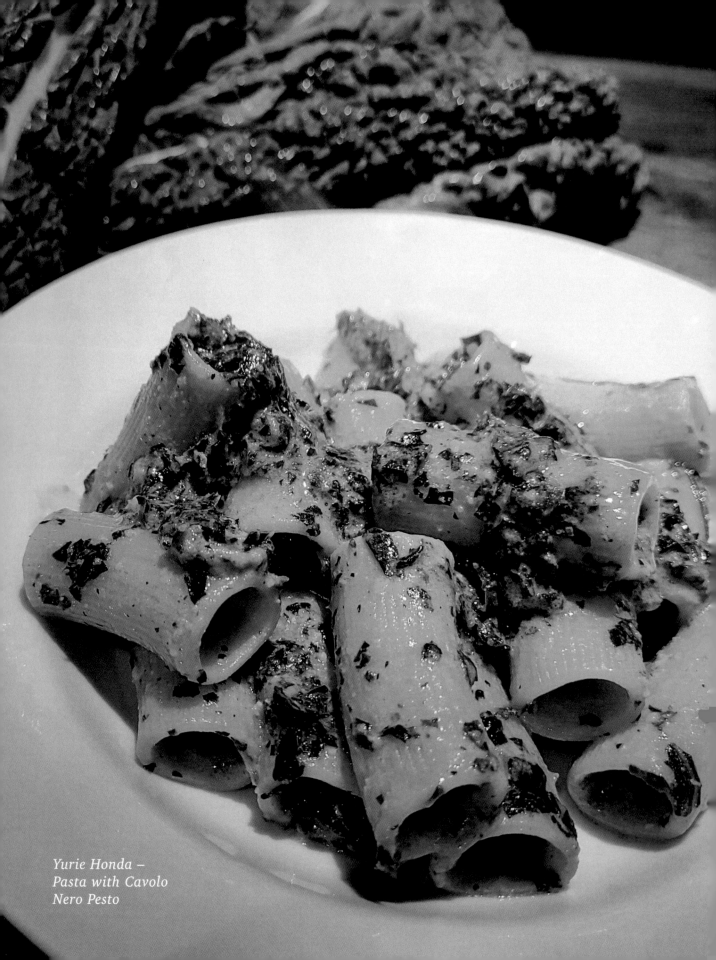

Yurie Honda –
Pasta with Cavolo
Nero Pesto

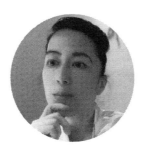

Yurie Honda
Japan & Italy

Yurie is a young chef who has trained and worked in Italy, bringing the best of Italian Mediterranean cuisine to her home city of Tokyo, Japan including as chef at Addu Mamma. Using local ingredients, including the possibility of Japanese Extra Virgin Olive Oil, she is frequently invited to demonstrate and teach at international shows and awards. Yurie is opening her new showcase restaurant in Tokyo in 2021.

Squid from the Pan

Serves: 4

Complexity:

Ingredients

800g of baby squid
320g of chopped tomatoes
2 cloves of garlic
4 tablespoons of Extra Virgin Olive Oil
Parsley to taste
Salt to taste
Pepper to taste

Method

1. Add 2 tablespoons of Extra Virgin Olive Oil to the pan with the sliced garlic.

2. Add the tomato, salt and pepper and cook for 10 min. Remove from the pan.

4. Wash and drain the squid and brown them for 5 minutes in the pan.

5. Pour the tomato sauce over the squid and cook for another 10-12min.

6. Sprinkle with chopped parsley. Serve hot.

Peperonata

Serves: 4

Complexity:

Ingredients

4 large peppers
400g of tomatoes
1 medium onion
8 of salted anchovies
1 tablespoon of salted capers
6 tablespoons of Extra Virgin Olive Oil

Method

1. Wash and dry the peppers, and clean the peppers from the seeds, then cut them into large pieces about 4-5cm.

2. Put the oil, the minced garlic, the minced onion, the anchovies, the salted capers in a pan.

3. Then add the peppers and tomatoes. Cook over low heat for 40 min. Bon appetit!

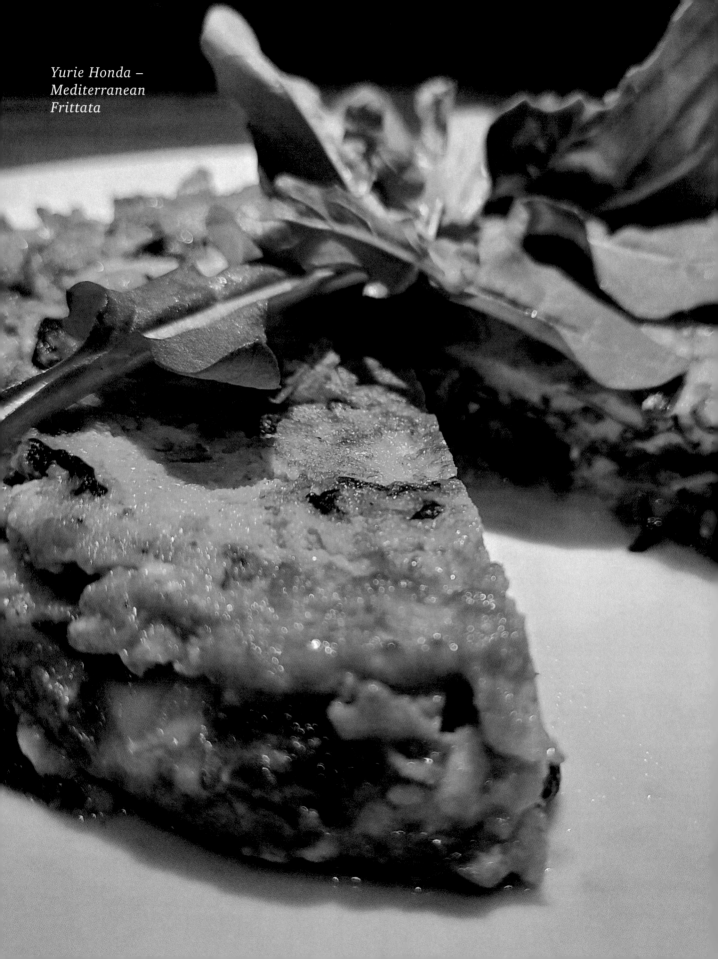

Yurie Honda –
Mediterranean
Frittata

Mediterranean Frittata

Serves: 1

Complexity:

Ingredients

4 eggs
120g mixed olives pitted (black olives and green olives)
60g mozzarella
1 bunch of rocket or chard
4 slices of anchovies in oil
4 tablespoons of Extra Virgin Olive Oil
Pinch of salt and pepper to taste

Method

1. Beat the eggs with the salt and pepper.

2. Chop the olives and then mix well.

3. Cut the mozzarella into 12 sticks

4. Wash and dry the rocket (or chard)

5. Cut the anchovy threads in half.

6. Put a non-stick pan on the heat and pour in 1/4 of the mixture. When the omelette is still soft, fill it with mozzarella, a few rocket leaves and halved anchovy fillets and add the remaining mixture.

7. Fold the sides and turn it to cook on the other side until all the ingredients are cooked. Enjoy your meal!

Carne alla Pizzaiola

Serves: 1

Complexity:

Ingredients

320g of lean cuts of beef, chicken, pork or lamb
200ml chopped tomatoes or passata with vegetable stock
1 clove of garlic
Mixed olives stones removed
2 tablespoons of Extra Virgin Olive Oil
Seasoning including Italian herbs such as oregano or rosemary, with a pinch of salt and pepper to taste
Grated Parmesan or Pecorino cheese

Method

1. Pour the oil into a pan, add the minced garlic and let it brown.

2. Add the tomato sauce and a little water or stock, add salt and pepper.

3. Cook for 10 minutes over medium heat, add the slices of beef and olives, cover with a lid and cook the meat*, turning the slices and adding the oregano.

4. Serve hot and with grated cheese, a sprig of basil and Extra Virgin Olive Oil. Enjoy your meal!

* Cooking time and amount of stock or added water will depend on the meat. Ensure chicken and pork in particular are fully cooked throughout.

Pasta with Cavolo Nero Pesto

Serves: 4

Complexity:

Ingredients

320g of pasta (spaghetti or linguine)
320g of cavolo nero
50g of almonds
50g of walnuts
80ml of Extra Virgin Olive Oil
40g of pecorino or parmesan cheese
1 clove of garlic
Pinch of salt and pepper

Method

1. Wash and dry the black cavolo nero leaves and remove the central and hard rib.

2. Blanch them in hot water for 5min.

3. Dry them very well.

4. In a chopper mixer, first grind the almonds and walnuts, minced garlic, cheese. Then add the cooked black cavolo nero leaves and Extra Virgin Olive Oil. Blend very well until a soft and creamy texture is achieved.

5. Throw the spaghetti into boiling, salted water, then drain them al dente and pour them into the pan together with the black cavolo nero pesto. Mix well.

6. Serve with a sprinkle of cheese and a drizzle of raw Extra Virgin Olive Oil. Enjoy your meal!

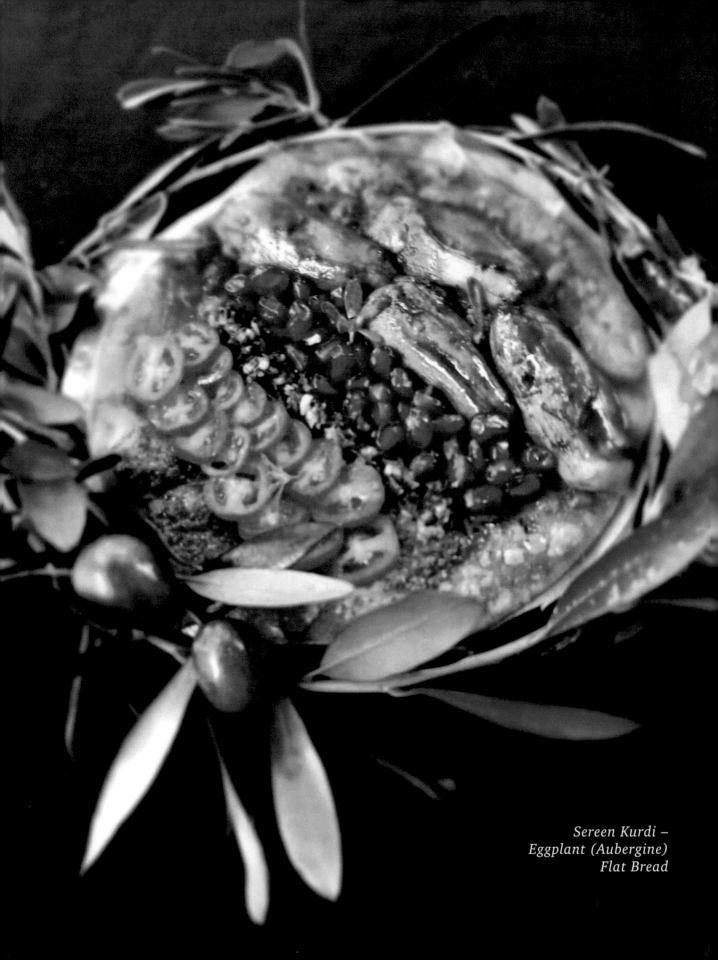

Sereen Kurdi –
Eggplant (Aubergine)
Flat Bread

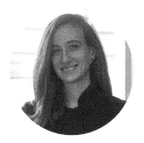

Sereen Kurdi
Jordan

After graduating with merit from Les Roches, Jordan, Sereen was awarded a full scholarship to study at Kendall College in Chicago. She graduated Summa Cum Laude and was then hired by Chef Marcus Jernmark of Aquavit in New York. She moved back to Amman, Jordan, and began teaching at the Royal Academy of Culinary Arts, before accepting a position as head chef for Her Majesty Queen Noor Al Hussein. In 2015, Kurdi founded The Local Table, Jordan's first pop-up dinner concept, focused on having a dinner fully sourced from local and organic products, while supporting local artisan food producers.

Eggplant (Aubergine) Flat Bread

Serves: 1

Complexity:

Flat Bread Recipe

¼ cup of whole wheat flour
⅛ cup of warm water
1 tbps Extra Virgin Olive Oil
⅛ tsp Dried or fresh wild thyme
Sprinkle of sea salt

Toppings

2 pc Baby eggplant
15g pomegranate seeds
1 tbsp Extra Virgin Olive Oil
1 tbsp Pomegranate molasses
¼ cup Fresh coriander leaves
3 cloves Garlic
¼ tsp Sea Salt
1/8 tsp Black pepper
5 pcs Cherry tomato

Method

For the flat bread

Add the flour, salt, thyme and ¾ tbsp Extra Virgin Olive Oil to a bowl and cut the fat into flour by rubbing it together.

Then add the water slowly and knead the dough until it comes together.

Add the rest of the Extra Virgin Olive Oil to a bowl and rest the dough covered for 30 minutes.

Roll the dough in a 1mm round.

Panfry the dough in a heated pan with Extra Virgin Olive Oil on both sides until crispy.

1. Char the eggplants on top of a gas stove or in the oven until the eggplant skin is charred

2. Chop the coriander leaves and mince the garlic

3. Peel the charred eggplants carefully and slice in half

4. Slice the cherry tomatoes

5. In a pan sweat the garlic and coriander in Extra Virgin Olive Oil with a bit of salt

6. Season the tomatoes with salt, pepper and Extra Virgin Olive Oil

7. Season the eggplant with pomegranate molasses, Extra Virgin Olive Oil and salt

8. Top the flat bread with all the topping and serve at room temperature

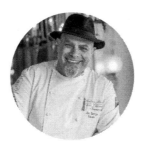

Joe Barza
Lebanon

Joe Barza, an international Master Celebrity Chef, is world-renowned for his specialization in Lebanese cuisine. With more than 30 years of professional cooking and kitchen management experience, Chef Joe proudly positions himself as the Lebanese Terroir Culinary Artist. In addition to being featured on major international media channels including CNN and *The New York Times*, Joe won the World Champion title for Tuna in Carlo Forte, Sardinia, and received many international recognitions and awards including but not limited to the Master Chef designation in 2010. He was also appointed as a jury member in many international culinary competitions and head judge in the Emmy Award-winning television show *Top Chef* in its Middle Eastern version in 2011.

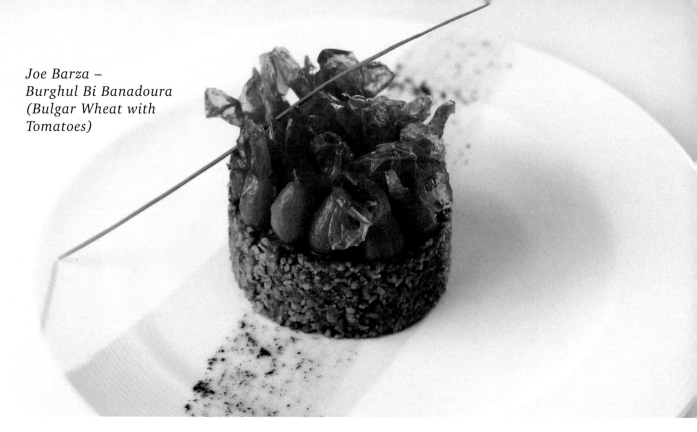

Joe Barza –
Burghul Bi Banadoura
(Bulgar Wheat with
Tomatoes)

Burghul Bi Banadoura (Bulgar Wheat with Tomatoes)

Serves: 4

Complexity: 🫗🫗

Ingredients

500g White coarse burghul
70g Extra Virgin Olive Oil
70g White onions, chopped
1 Garlic clove, finely chopped
1.5 L Peeled tomatoes, chopped
50g Tomato paste
12g Salt
5g Allspice powder
150g Water

Garnish

200 g Cherry tomatoes
Fresh Chives

Method

1. Wash the burghul and drain very well.

2. Keep aside.

3. In a pot, heat the Extra Virgin Olive Oil on high heat.

4. Add the onions and sauté until translucent.

5. Add the garlic and stir for 1 minute.

6. Add the burghul and stir for 3 minutes.

7. Add in the peeled tomatoes and the tomato paste and season with salt and pepper.

8. Add the water and lower the heat. Let it simmer for 20 min over low heat with the lid on until the bulgur is well cooked.

Cherry tomato preparation

With the edge of a sharp knife slice a shallow X into the bottom of the tomato.

Bring a pot of water to boil and place the tomatoes into the water.

Blanch the tomatoes for 5 seconds. You should be able to pop them out of their skins by giving them a twist and squeeze.

Plate dressing

In a plate fill in the burghul preparation in a circle mold.

Garnish with the cherry tomatoes and the chives.

Serve and enjoy.

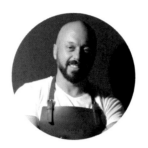

Charbel Safi
Lebanon

Charbel Safi is a name that became a sensation in the culinary world in a short period of time. In a field where being a spectacular chef has become a harder challenge to achieve, he was able to mark his own territory fusing creativity and cutting-edge techniques resulting in unprecedented inventions. From a young age, Charbel Safi has been climbing the ladder of success one milestone after the other. After studying culinary art in Lebanon, he took his passion further all the way to Paris, France, where he trained in one of the most famous 3-Michelin star restaurants. Equipped with the masterful knowledge of international cuisine, he took on the role of Executive Chef of Faqra Club, one of the leading resorts in the country, aged just 23.

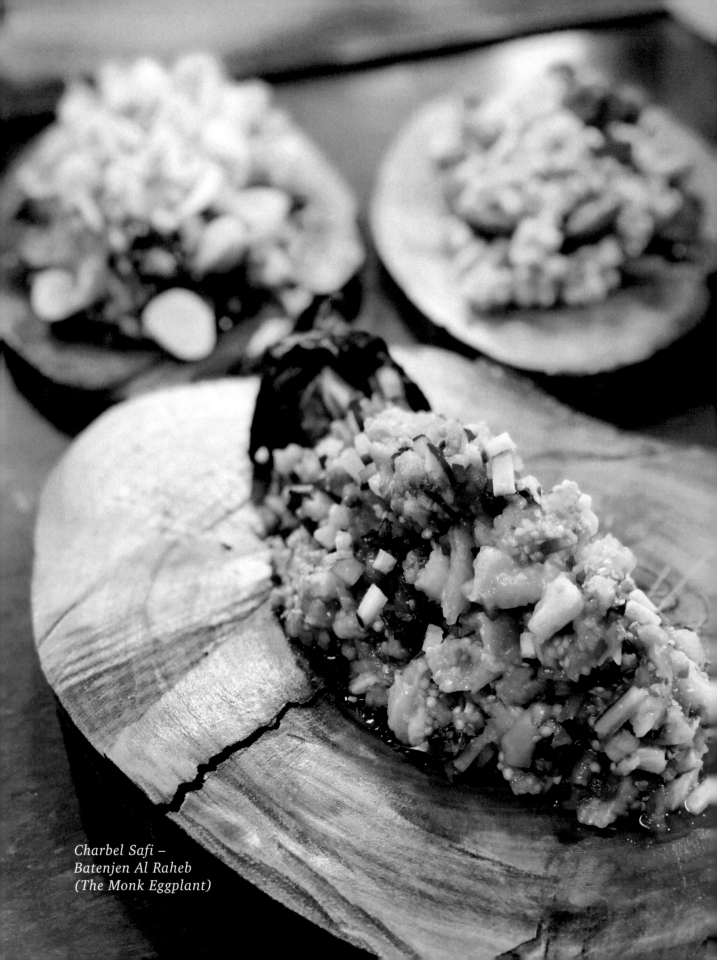

Charbel Safi –
Batenjen Al Raheb
(The Monk Eggplant)

Batenjen Al Raheb (The Monk Eggplant)

Batenjen al Raheb is an old recipe based on hand picked organic vegetables from the Lebanese mountains. This dish used as Lebanese cold mezze, healthy and well-known as a vegan dish, especially during fasting season.

Serves: 1

Complexity:

Ingredients

Eggplant	1pc 600g
Diced onion	50g
Diced green capsicum	50g
Diced cucumber	50g
Diced radish	30g
Diced tomato skin	30g
Chopped parsley	5g
Chopped mint	3 leaves
Extra Virgin Olive Oil	50ml
Lemon juice	30ml
Salt	5g
White pepper	pinch

Method

1. Prepare a hardwood charcoal fire in a grill.

2. Place eggplant directly on coals and cook, turning occasionally, until the skins are blackened.

3. Cook for around 10 minutes.

4. Transfer to a strainer and let cool slightly.

5. Carefully remove skin from eggplant.

Serving

Transfer peeled eggplant to a cutting board and cut into thick chunks but keep the stem on a side for plating presentation.

Combine egg plant with the vegetables, lemon juice and Extra Virgin Olive Oil, season with salt and white pepper.

Served cold on a wooden tray.

Roasted Chicken Whole Green Wheat

Serves: 4

Complexity: 🫙🫙🫙

Ingredients

Chicken Marinade

Boneless whole chicken 800g
Yogurt 2 tbsp
White grape vinegar 30g
Turmeric powder 5g
White ground pepper 1g
Fresh thyme leaves 3g
Cilantro leaves 3g
Basil leaves 3g
Extra Virgin Olive Oil 50ml

Method

1. Blend all ingredients together in an electric blender until the mixture becomes smooth and creamy.

2. Place boneless chicken in a flat tray skin side in the bottom, then cover with marinade.

3. Cover well and keep in fridge at least 2 hours. The Lebanese yogurt gives chicken or any meat more tenderness and a pleasantly sour taste.

4. Place whole chicken in a roasting pan.

5. Preheat oven to 160 degrees Celsius and bake for 45 minutes or according to instructions with the portion. Every 10 minutes brush the marinade mixture onto the chicken to keep the chicken juicy and tender and ensure fully cooked.

Whole Green Wheat

Whole green wheat 2cups
Vegetable stock 5cups
Diced onion 300g
Extra Virgin Olive Oil 30ml
Cumin powder 1sp
Caraway powder 2sp
Salt 5g
Green beans 400g
Leeks 1 stick

Method

1. Soak green wheat in water overnight.

2. Add oil to skillet, and stir in the diced onion. Cook for one minute.

3. Add soaked green wheat, stirring to coat with oil and onion.

4. Add spices and salt the cover with vegetable stock. Bring to a boil then cover and cook on low heat for 45 minutes.

6. Before serving always make sure that wheat is still juicy and always glazed with vegetable stock and spices, as with risotto.

Beans

1. Boil beans in water and pinch of salt for only 1minute. Remove and strain.

2. Cut leeks into belt shapes and boil in the same water for 30 seconds.

3. Divide beans into bunches of about 8 pieces, and roll with leek belts.

Toppings

Diced Indian onion 100g
Green leeks julienne 50g

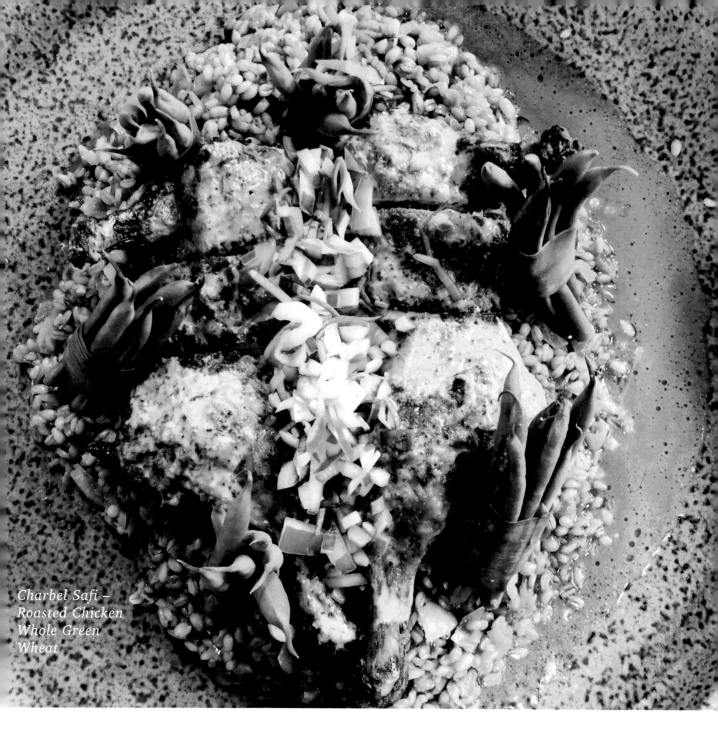

Charbel Safi –
Roasted Chicken
Whole Green
Wheat

Serving

1. Place cooked green wheat on a serving plate.

2. Cut whole roasted chicken into 6 pieces and serve over the wheat.

3. Decorate with green beans, chopped onion and leeks julienne.

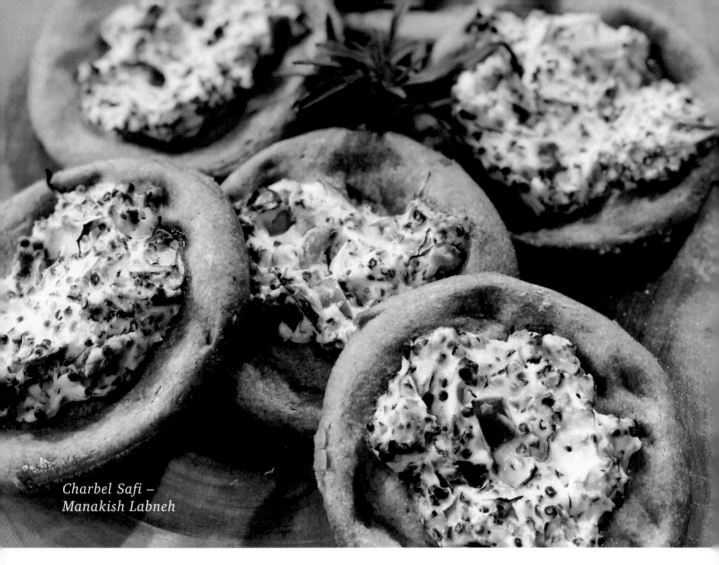

*Charbel Safi –
Manakish Labneh*

Manakish Labneh

Serves: 4

Complexity:

Ingredients

Whole Wheat Dough

Whole wheat flour	500g
Water	300ml
Fresh yeast	10g
Extra Virgin Olive Oil	50ml
Salt	10g

Labneh Filling

Labneh cheese	400g
Green olives diced	100g
Red quinoa boiled	100g
Tomato skin	50g
Fresh thyme julienne	2g
Mint leaves julienne	3g
Extra Virgin Olive Oil	50ml

Method

Labneh

Combine all ingredients together.

Dough

1. Combine yeast, water and Extra Virgin Olive Oil and stir well until dissolved. Allow to sit for 10 minutes until foam is formed on the top as result of yeast being activated.

2. In a large mixing bowl or stand mixer sift the flour with salt, add yeast mixture until a smooth dough is formed. Place in a bowl, cover and place in the fridge to rise (2 hours cold proofing)

3. Once ready punch down the dough and cut into 30g form balls.

4. Dust a clean work surface with flour, using your hand or rolling pin roll out the dough 5mm thick.

5. Place dough on an oven tray, add labneh mix on the top.

Serving

Bake in preheated oven 180 degrees Celsius for 10 minutes until golden around the edges and the bottom.

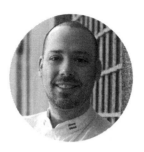

Daniel Garcia Peinado
Spain

Daniel García Peinado is an acclaimed chef throughout Spain and beyond. In addition to cooking and gastronomy, he has studied tourism, nutrition and dietetics. His cuisine is based on Extra Virgin Olive Oil and he is known as "The Chef of Extra Virgin Olive Oil" for his research work involving recommendations for cooking with Extra Virgin Olive Oil with the Universities of Granada and Cordoba.

He is currently a gastronomic consultant, executive chef of La Cala in Mijas and the Gourmet de la Roja initiative in association with the Spanish national football team. He is captain of the Spanish National Professional Chefs Team, having represented Spain and achieved fourth place in the Global Chefs Challenge. He has been a Spanish culinary ambassador, cooking for President Obama and the US Congress. He has worked with the Monell Institute and the Mayo Clinic promoting the correct use of Extra Virgin Olive Oil in diets and cooking styles.

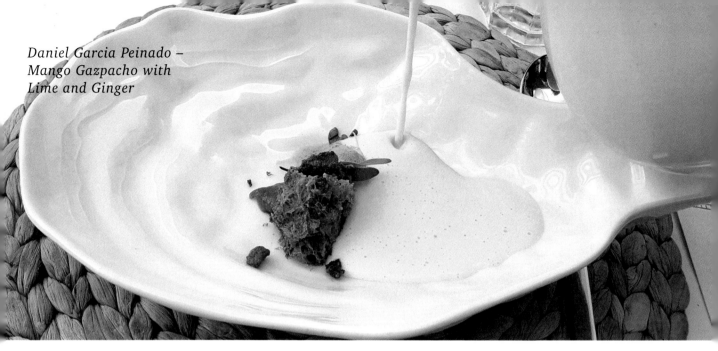

Mango Gazpacho with Lime and Ginger

Serves: 4

Complexity:

Ingredients

500g Mango purée
350ml Extra Virgin Olive Oil
1 litre water
75g ginger
50g green pepper
80g bread
3 limes
5g salt

Method

1. Add to blender the bread, Extra Virgin Olive Oil, limes, salt and 100g of purée.

2. Allow the bread to hydrate and grind to create a smooth paste.

3. Add ginger, pepper and the rest of the purée and pouring water, season and adjust the texture. Strain and serve cold.

Simple Olive and Anchovy Tapenade

Serves: 2-4

Complexity:

Ingredients

100 grams of black olives
35 grams of capers
45 grams of anchovies
150ml of Hojiblanca Extra Virgin Olive Oil

Method

Grind all ingredients except Extra Virgin Olive Oil using a blender, then add and mix Extra Virgin Olive Oil, serve cold.

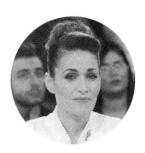

Ahlem Nguili
Tunisia & France

Born in Paris, originally from beautiful Tunisia, Ahlem began her career as a lawyer but kept her love for cooking throughout the years and followed her dream to train as a chef.

For almost 12 years, cooking has been everything for her – "It's a sweet obsession" as she says. She is an active member of the illustrious chefs' association Toques Françaises, having studied at the traditional "Sœurs Brettonnes de St Merri". And with a passionate grandmother who introduced her to the most authentic Tunisian cuisine from an early age, Ahlem brings the flavours of North Africa to everything she does. She is an international consulting chef and currently works in Paris.

Slata Mechwya – A Tradition of Tunisia

Serves: 2-4

Complexity:

Ingredients

600g of fresh red tuna*
60g boutarga powder where available
400g green peppers
200g of red peppers
1 chilli
400g Roma tomatoes
200g eggplants
200g small size onions
1 garlic clove

Sesame
Harissa spices
Salt and pepper
Caraway powder
Juice of half a lemon
Dried mint
Extra Virgin Olive Oil
Young almonds
Small Basque peppers

Method

1. Marinate the tuna strips in the harissa.

2. Grill the vegetables until very pronounced coloring of the skin.

3. Place the vegetables in a plastic bag to obtain condensation in order to easily remove their skin, leave at least 40 minutes.

4. Peel the vegetables and crush them with a mortar.

5. Season the salad with salt, pepper, caraway, lemon juice Extra Virgin Olive Oil and dried mint.

6. Garnish the tataki with sesame and cut.

7. Dress the salad, not forgetting your dash of boutarga, almonds, the pretty Basque peppers and anoint the dish with a drizzle of Extra Virgin Olive Oil.

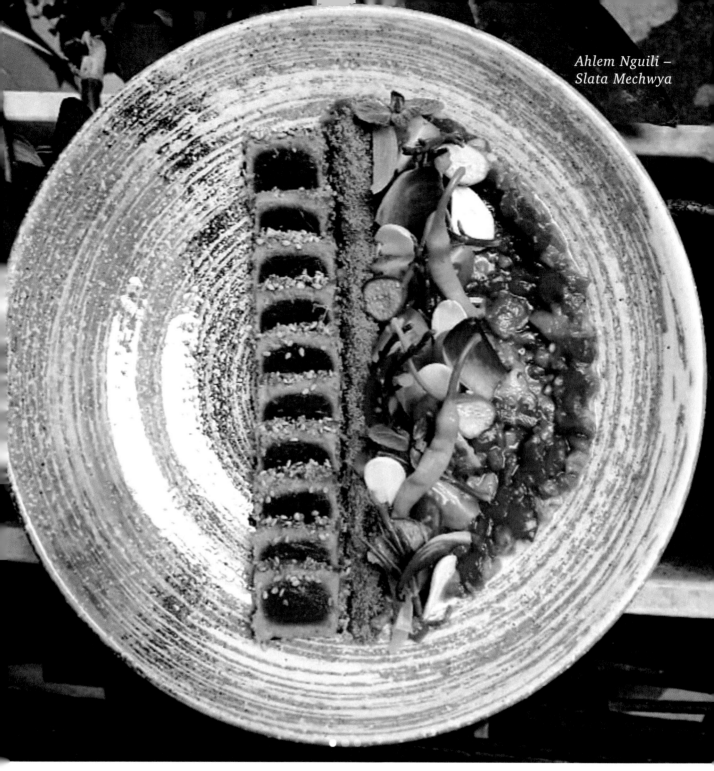

Ahlem Nguili –
Slata Mechwya

* Please note – Ahlem and other chefs creating sushi or carpaccio dishes are skilled in selecting and preparing raw food safely. When consuming raw or lightly cooked fish, it is always recommended to following public health recommendations and ensure it is suitable and safe for consumption.

175

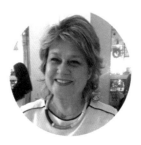

Ilknur Turkeli Civelek
Turkey

Following a career as an economist, Ilknur pursued her ambition to learn more about the plants and herbs of her native Turkey and their nutritional importance, gaining degrees in Agriculture and Culinary Arts. Growing up on the Aegean coast of Anatolia amongst ancient olive groves led her to become a certified Olive Oil sommelier and technical taster. She currently conducts masterclasses and is a consultant on the subject of the Mediterranean lifestyle, specialising in Olive Oil tasting and its use in cooking. Here she presents a typical sweet cake with Extra Virgin Olive Oil, consumed on special occasions.

Lemon Cakes with Extra Virgin Olive Oil

Serves: 2-4

Complexity:

Ingredients

165g flour
2 eggs
75g powder sugar
Zest of a lemon
1 table spoon lemon juice
1 tea spoon baking powder
60 ml Extra Virgin Olive Oil

Method

1. Preheat to oven to 190 Centigrade.

2. Beat the eggs and the sugar for about 5-7 minutes.

3. Add the lemon juice and the zest and lightly stir with a spatula.

4. Add half of the Extra Virgin Olive Oil and stir. Add half of the flour and baking powder and stir. Add the rest of the oil and rest of the flour whilst stirring. Rest the mix about 6-7 minutes.

5. Place the mix into small silicon moulds or cup-cakes. Bake about 10-12 minutes. Always check with a toothpick to see if the cakes are baked since cooking time can vary from oven to oven.

6. Serving luke warm is recommended. Extra Virgin Olive Oil with a mild aroma is recommended.

Omelette with Fresh Tomatoes and Peppers

Serves: 2

Complexity:

Ingredients

2 Peppers (Bell or Chili)
3 ripe tomatoes
5 eggs
2 spoons Extra Virgin Olive Oil
Salt
Black Pepper

Method

1. Cut peppers fine julienne and grate the tomatoes.

2. Sautée peppers in Extra Virgin Olive Oil over medium heat on pan.

3. Add the grated tomatoes, when peppers are softened and cook them together until the mix come to a certain consistency.

4. Lower the heat, add the eggs and stir lightly. Done in few minutes.

Green Beans in Extra Virgin Olive Oil

Serves: 2-4

Complexity:

Ingredients

1 kg green beans (Romano, roller beans or alike), strings removed cut lengthwise, if needed
2 medium onions (fine sliced, julienne)
2 garlic cloves, finely sliced
4 medium size tomatoes, peeled and cut fine, diced
Salt
Black pepper
3 table spoons of Extra Virgin Olive Oil

Method

1. Sautee the onions and garlic in a pot about 5 min over medium heat. Do not caramelize, just sweat them.

2. Then add the beans, stir them well and make sure they are all covered with Extra Virgin Olive Oil and onion mix.

3. Add the tomatoes, salt, pepper and stir and cook about 5 min. Add hot water until water covers the beans.

4. Cook for an additional 30 minutes over medium heat until the beans are soft. Remove the heat and get it chilled down about 10 min. minimum. Best eaten at room temperature. A little sprinkle of raw Extra Virgin Olive Oil after cooling makes it shine and adds wonderful green aromas, which can be lost during cooking because of heat. Arbequina or Koroneiki of the harvest year or an Extra Virgin Olive Oil with higher polyphenol levels of previous harvest year with green aromas is recommended.

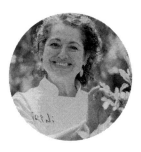

Irini Tzortzoglou
United Kingdom & Crete

Irini was born in a small village in Crete in Greece in 1958, moved with her family to Athens for her education and in 1980 to London with her first husband who was English. She worked in banking in the City of London for over 30 years, but retired early in order to spend more time in Crete, and with her second husband John moved to the Lake District in 2010. Always connected to her rich heritage and passionate about food, Irini competed and won *MasterChef* in 2019. In January 2020 Irini became an Olive Oil sommelier and her first book, *Under the Olive Tree (recipes from my Greek kitchen)* was published by Headline in July 2020.

Sunshine salad of golden beetroot, orange and fennel

A warm purple beetroot salad has been a family staple for as long as I can remember. The beetroots, like so many other vegetables, were so sweet and full of flavour that the only treatment was to boil them (I am not sure about that way of cooking anything, as so much is lost to the water), peel them and toss them in good Extra Virgin Olive Oil and red wine vinegar. The stalks were always used too.

In this salad I am using golden beetroots, as their sweetness is reminiscent of the purple ones of home – whatever flavour shortfall there is, the aromatic, zingy citrus dressing addresses it perfectly.

Once again, I would advocate roasting the beetroots with aromatics. Concentrating their flavour is paramount, and helping this delicious root vegetable lose some of its liquid by cooking it dry will do just that.

The number of beetroots is based on the fact that they tend to generally be on the small size, but it is best you judge how many you need. Being a Greek, I believe it is always better to have leftovers and eat them the next day than be short of anything, particularly when entertaining!

Serves: 4

Complexity:

Ingredients

A handful of pistachio nuts
4–5 golden beetroots, preferably with their stalks
Extra Virgin Olive Oil, for drizzling
a sprig of fresh thyme
2 garlic cloves, unpeeled
2 oranges
1 packet of watercress
2 baby gem lettuces
½ a fennel bulb, fronds reserved

For the beetroot stalks

1 tbsp Extra Virgin Olive Oil
A squeeze of lemon juice
For the dressing
300ml freshly squeezed orange juice
zest of 1 unwaxed orange
20ml lemon juice
1 tsp orange blossom honey
50ml Extra Virgin Olive Oil
seeds from 3 cardamom pods, crushed
1cm piece of fresh ginger, peeled and grated

Method

1. Preheat the oven to 180°C/350°F/gas 4. Roast the pistachios on a baking tray for 5–7 minutes, then put aside to cool.

2. Cut the stalks off the beetroots and set aside. Wash and dry the beetroots and place them on a piece of foil large enough to wrap them completely. Drizzle with a little oil, season with salt and pepper, then add the sprig of thyme and the garlic cloves, wrap well and place in the oven. Check for tenderness after 1 hour by inserting a knife, though they may need as long as 1½ hours, depending on their size.

3. Wash the stalks and cut them into pieces about 5cm long. Drop them into a pan of boiling water with a pinch of salt and cook for a few minutes, until soft but still with a bit of crunch, then drain and rinse under cold water. Put them into a bowl with a drizzle of oil and a squeeze of lemon, and season.

4. Take the beetroots out of the oven when cooked and leave to cool. Peel, thinly slice and put into a bowl. Drizzle with a little oil and season with salt and pepper.

5. Peel the oranges and divide into segments, discarding the membrane. Rinse and drain the watercress. Trim the ends off the lettuces and slice them horizontally into ½ cm-thick rings. With a vegetable peeler or a mandolin, shave the fennel.

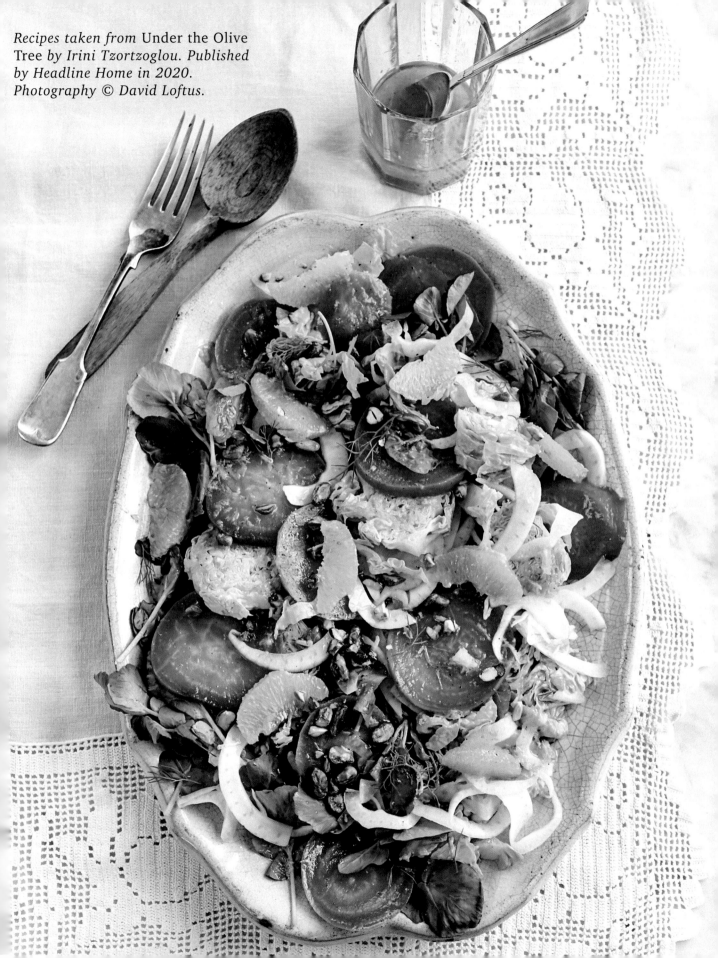

6. To make the dressing, bring the orange juice and zest to the boil in a small saucepan, then boil until reduced by half. Place in a small blender and add the lemon juice, honey, oil and a pinch of salt and pepper, and blend to a thick consistency. Add the cardamom seeds and grated ginger and give it a good stir.

7. On a flat serving plate, arrange the beetroot slices, watercress, fennel shavings, orange segments and baby gem slices in layers, scattering some of the beetroot stalks here and there. Drizzle the dressing over the salad and scatter over the roasted pistachios and fennel fronds.

Roast chicken with root vegetables and chickpea salad

More than anything else, I love chicken for its versatility. It is the blank canvas of all meats for me. We always had our own chickens in Crete, and although the flavour of the meat and eggs does not compare with anything I have eaten outside the island since, the aroma of chicken roasting always takes me back to a very happy place. These days I content myself with Aunty Antonia's home-grown chicken, which she cooks for me every time I visit.

Supermarket chicken can still taste delicious, though, and John and I always fight for the crispy chicken skin. Being just the two of us means that, when roasting a whole chicken, we can make three meals from it, the first being the freshly roasted legs with accompanying roast vegetables, the second the breasts in a salad the following day, as here, and the third a chicken, egg and lemon soup made from the carcass.

Serves: 4

Complexity:

Ingredients

2 carrots, cut into 1cm-thick slices
2 peppers, de-seeded and cut into large square pieces
2 courgettes, cut into 2cm-thick slices or 6–8 whole baby courgettes
2 medium onions, quartered
3 garlic cloves, peeled but left whole
Extra Virgin Olive Oil, for drizzling
A sprig of fresh thyme, leaves picked
A handful of baby plum tomatoes, cut in half
500ml water
150g bulgur
1 x 400g tin of chickpeas
2 tbsp finely chopped fresh parsley
Zest of 1 unwaxed lemon
2 roasted chicken breasts

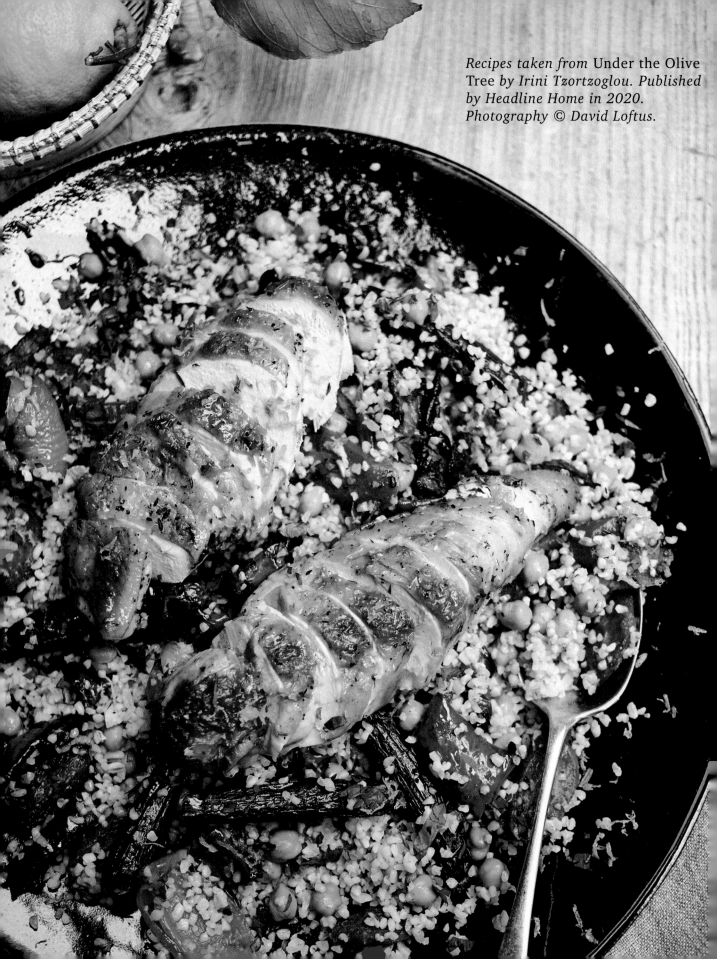

Recipes taken from Under the Olive Tree *by Irini Tzortzoglou. Published by Headline Home in 2020. Photography © David Loftus.*

Method

1. Preheat the oven to 180°C/350°F/gas 4.

2. Place the carrots, peppers, courgettes, onions and garlic in a roasting tray. Sprinkle with oil, scatter over the thyme leaves and season with salt and pepper. Bake for 20 minutes, then add the tomatoes. Continue baking for another 20 minutes, or until the vegetables are soft and caramelised.

3. In a saucepan bring the water to the boil with a pinch of salt and add the bulgur. Let it cook for 10–15 minutes, until it's soft and plump. Drain, then put it back into the saucepan and cover.

4. Drain and rinse the chickpeas. Toss with the bulgur and the roasted vegetables, and add the parsley and lemon zest. Check the seasoning. Serve on a platter, topped with the sliced chicken breasts.

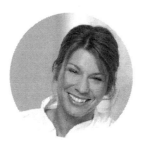

Maria Elia
United Kingdom & Cyprus

Maria knew she wanted to be a chef at the age of four, citing her father's Cypriot restaurant as a source of inspiration. Progressing through the culinary world and a rigorous apprenticeship in London including stages at El Bulli and Arzak, Maria then made a name for herself heading up the kitchens at Delfina and Whitechapel Gallery Dining Room. Head-hunted to open a restaurant at a five-star boutique resort in California, Maria created a unique fresh and eclectic Greek Californian cuisine which gained rave reviews.

After spending time in Rwanda running a successful Supper Club business Maria is now based in the UK where she writes, cooks and teaches and has established herself as a consultant in demand, designing concepts for restaurant start-ups and various projects around the globe. She is the author of 3 award-winning books: *The Modern Vegetarian*, *Full of Flavour* and *Smashing Plates* which draws on her Anglo Greek heritage-redefining Greek cuisine as we know it! In between projects Maria can be found at various pop ups, where she combines influences from her Greek heritage with the best of British produce to give an eclectic mix of Greek flavours and ingredients.

Fassoulaki 'Ladera'
Green Beans Braised in Extra Virgin Olive Oil

Serves: 4

Complexity:

Ingredients

100ml Extra Virgin Olive Oil
900g of runner beans (or green beans if out of season)
1 large onion, finely chopped
2 cloves garlic, finely chopped
2 potatoes/1 large, cut into 2cm chunks (optional)
3 ripe vine tomatoes, grated (or 400g tin tomatoes, chopped)
1 teaspoon sugar
1 small bunch parsley, finely chopped

Method

1. Trim and wash the green beans, then heat the Extra Virgin Olive Oil in a large pot over a medium heat.

2. Add the onion and cook until softened and without colour, add the garlic, beans and potatoes and cook for a further 6 minutes stirring to coat in the Extra Virgin Olive Oil.

3. Add the tomatoes, sugar and season with sea salt and pepper.

4. Add just enough hot water to half cover the beans and potatoes, cover and simmer over a low heat for approximately 35-40 minutes until the sauce has reduced and clings to the tender beans.

5. Stir in the parsley and serve drizzled with Greek Extra Virgin Olive Oil, 'Ladera' beans are best eaten warm as opposed to hot. Delicious served with crusty bread and topped with crumbled feta or served with little lemon juice squeezed over the top.

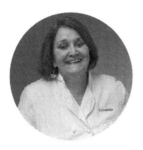

Valentina Harris
United Kingdom & Italy

Valentina Harris is the noted authority on Italian food and food culture and a member of the International Association of Culinary Professionals. Descending from the important Renaissance Sforza family, Valentina is bright, passionate, accessible and appeals to people far beyond her chosen subject. Being a prolific author as well as doing many TV appearances, she is always in demand to appear at top food events. She has given innumerable live cookery demonstrations and lectures extensively across Europe, Australia, New Zealand, Japan and South Africa.

Valentina's first cookery book, *Perfect Pasta*, has been translated into six languages and won The Award for Literature and Gastronomy in Germany. Seven other books followed on from the success of *Perfect Pasta* culminating in the BBC six-part television series titled *Italian Regional Cookery*. Valentina is now established as a prolific writer on Italian food and cuisine and regularly features on television and radio and contributes to many leading national newspapers and magazines.

La Puttanesca

This famous and much loved sauce is named for the ladies of the night of Rome. By which I mean that it needs to be gutsy and potent! You should be able to taste all the different ingredients in the sauce individually.

Serves: 4

Complexity:

Ingredients

1 to 2 cloves garlic, finely chopped, or cut in half, or whole - crushed or uncrushed
8 tablespoons Extra Virgin Olive Oil
3–5 anchovy fillets (either salted or canned in oil, rinsed and dried)
1 to 4 small dried red chilli peppers, chopped finely
1 tablespoon rinsed and dried salted capers, roughly chopped
200 g (6 oz)/1 cup canned chopped tomatoes
Very large pinch dried oregano
Sea salt and freshly milled black pepper
1/2 cup (120 mls) (4 fl. oz) dry white wine
Handful of de-stoned black olives (N.B. a black olive that is sold without a stone is a green olive that has been de-stoned and then dyed. So unless the black olives in a jar look really beaten up and scruffy avoid at all costs – it is not possible to de-stone a soft and ripe black olive without damageing it! Buy them with a stone and then do the de-stoning yourself.)
Handful of fresh flat leaf parsley, roughly chopped

Method

1. Very gently, without burning, fry the garlic and half the oil together with the anchovy fillets and the dried chilli pepper, until the anchovy dissolves into the oil.

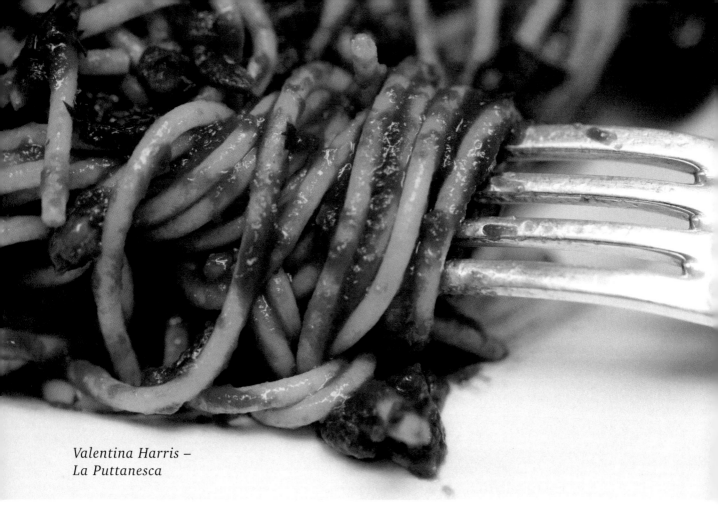

Valentina Harris –
La Puttanesca

2. Add the capers and the tomatoes and stir together thoroughly. Simmer for a few minutes, and then add the oregano, seasoning, wine and olives.

3. Stir and leave to simmer gently for at least 15 minutes, though if longer, it does no harm.

4. Serve over freshly cooked pasta, traditionally penne or spaghetti, tossed together with the remaining Extra Virgin Olive Oil and a generous handful of freshly chopped flat leaf parsley.

Tip: You can vary the intensity of heat and overall flavour by reducing or increasing the amount of garlic and chilli in the sauce. If you are not chopping the garlic, do remember to remove the larger whole or halved garlic clove either before adding the tomatoes or before tossing the sauce with the pasta.

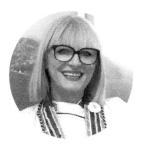

Maria Loi
United States & Greece

Chef Maria Loi is an internationally renowned entrepreneur, author, television personality and philanthropist working to change the world – one healthy bite at a time. Known as the Julia Child of Greece, she is the founder and face of a lifestyle brand that nurtures a healthy body and soul, melds the inspiration of ancient Greece with a modern approach to the Mediterranean diet, cooks up a heaping dose of happiness, humor and joy and helps people boost their immunity and improve their health, wellness and longevity.

Chef Loi is passionate about sharing the magic of all things Greek – especially the culinary treasures, recipes and practices passed down through the generations and from her grandfather. Deeply popular and beloved in Greece and a food superstar in the U.S., she exudes kindness, friendliness and warmth, makes a friend of everyone she meets and lights up rooms with her bountiful energy, infectious smile and hearty laugh.

The namesake of three restaurants, including the current Loi Estiatorio in Manhattan, Chef Loi has cooked for celebrities and Presidents. But she most enjoys gathering with a roomful of diners over a good meal filled with laughter and stories and passing out smiles and homemade cookies to children who visit her restaurant. Named an official Ambassador of Greek Gastronomy by the Chef's Club of Greece, Chef Loi is also a passionate and dedicated philanthropist who supports a wide variety of causes focused on children and the underserved.

Fasolia Salata
Greek White Bean Salad

Serves: 4-6

Complexity:

Ingredients

1 pound (450g) dried cannellini beans
1 white onion, halved
1 teaspoon salt
1/3 cup Greek Extra Virgin Olive Oil
1 medium red onions, finely chopped
1 green bell pepper, finely chopped
1 bunch scallions, finely chopped
1 bunch fresh dill, chopped
1-2 medium tomatoes, finely chopped
2 oz Feta cheese
Salt and freshly ground black pepper

Dressing
1/3 cup red wine vinegar
2/3 cup Greek Extra Virgin Olive Oil
Salt and freshly ground black pepper
Greek Oregano

Method

1. The night before you plan to serve this dish, place the beans in a large bowl with water to cover by 2 or 3 inches. Set aside to soak overnight.

2. The next day, drain the beans into a colander and discard the soaking liquid. Place the beans and halved onion (both halves) in a large pot, add water to cover; add a teaspoon of salt and 2/3 cup of Greek Extra Virgin Olive Oil, bring to a boil and cook until beans are fairly soft, about 35-40 minutes. Remove

the beans from the heat and drain them into a large colander, discarding the cooking liquid. Rinse the beans well and drain them again. Allow to cool for half hour, then rinse under cold water, and drain again. Reserve.

3. Add the red onions, green pepper, scallions, dill, and tomatoes to a large mixing bowl; add the cooked beans, and toss gently to combine. Taste, and season accordingly with salt and pepper.

4. To make the dressing, combine 1/3 cup of red wine vinegar with 2/3 cup of Extra Virgin Olive Oil in a resealable container, and season with salt, pepper, and Greek oregano to taste. Shake vigorously until emulsified.

5. Dress the salad with as little or as much dressing as preferred, tossing gently to fully combine; crumble the feta into the salad, and toss again to fully combine. Serve and enjoy!

Cook's Notes: Tailor this recipe to your taste! Use different beans, or additional varieties; use your favorite herbs, vegetables, and seasonings to make this recipe your own – remember, if you don't like something, change it!

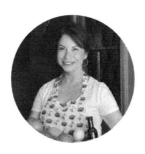

Amy Riolo
United States & Italy

As an award-winning, best-selling author, chef, television personality, cuisine and culture expert, and educator, Amy Riolo is known for sharing history, culture, and nutrition through global cuisine. A graduate of Cornell University, Amy is considered one of the world's foremost authorities on culinary culture. She is a culinary thought leader who enjoys changing the way we think about food and the people who create it.

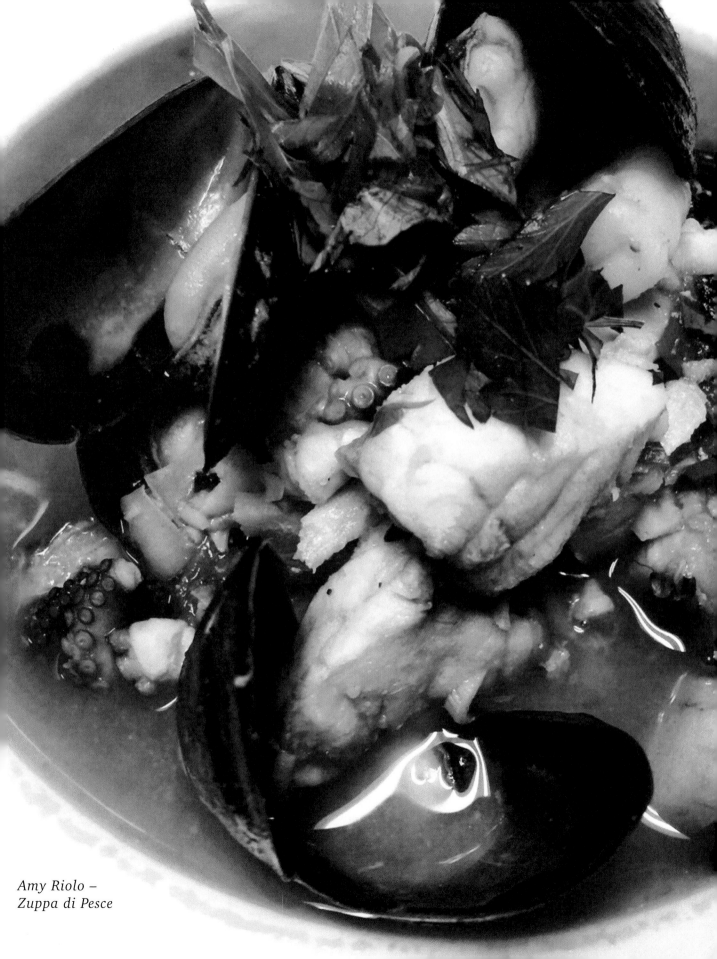

Amy Riolo –
Zuppa di Pesce

Zuppa di Pesce
Italian Seafood Soup

One of my favorite memories in my ancestral hometown of Crotone, Italy is going to the marina to buy seafood with my cousin Angela. After picking up the freshest choices possible from the sparkling Ionian Sea, we then head back to her home to cook. In Italy, as in other places in the Mediterranean region, seafood that is not caught that day is not considered fresh.

Each Italian coastal region has their own variation of this stew. When making fish soup, local fishermen would traditionally use the fish left behind after more valuable fish have sold. Use your favorite seafood combination to come up with the version of this dish you like best.

Serves: 8

Complexity:

Ingredients

1/4 cup Extra Virgin Olive Oil
1 tablespoon minced parsley
1/2 teaspoon crushed red chile flakes
Pinch of good-quality saffron
5 cloves garlic, minced
12 ounces calamari, cleaned and cut into 1-inch pieces
12 ounces baby octopus, cleaned, and cut into 1-inch pieces, if desired
1 cup dry white wine
2 cups chopped fresh tomatoes, juice reserved
1/4 teaspoon freshly ground black pepper
1 cup Homemade Seafood Stock or water
1 (1-pound) mullet or other white fish fillet, cut into 2-inch pieces
12 ounces large shell-on shrimp
12 ounces mussels, scrubbed and debearded

Method

1. Heat oil in a 6-quart saucepan over medium heat. Add parsley, saffron, chile flakes, and minced garlic, and cook until fragrant, about 1 minute. Add calamari and octopus and cook, stirring occasionally, until seafood is opaque, about 4 minutes. Add wine and cook, stirring often, until the liquid has evaporated, about 20 minutes.

2. Add tomatoes along with their juice, season with pepper, and cook, stirring occasionally, until seafood is tender, about 10 minutes. Stir in stock, cover, and simmer for 10 minutes.

3. Add monkfish and cook, covered, until fish is just firm, about 5 minutes. Add mullet and shrimp to the pot, and scatter mussels over top. Cook, covered, without stirring (so as not to break up the seafood), until the mullet is just cooked through and the mussels have just opened, about 10 minutes.

4. Ladle stew into bowls and serve.

COOKING CONVERSION CHART

Measurement

CUP	ONCES	MILLILITERS	TABLESPOONS
8 cup	64 oz	1895 ml	128
6 cup	48 oz	1420 ml	96
5 cup	40 oz	1180 ml	80
4 cup	32 oz	960 ml	64
2 cup	16 oz	480 ml	32
1 cup	8 oz	240 ml	16
3/4 cup	6 oz	177 ml	12
2/3 cup	5 oz	158 ml	11
1/2 cup	4 oz	118 ml	8
3/8 cup	3 oz	90 ml	6
1/3 cup	2.5 oz	79 ml	5.5
1/4 cup	2 oz	59 ml	4
1/8 cup	1 oz	30 ml	3
1/16 cup	1/2 oz	15 ml	1

Temperature

FAHRENHEIT	CELSIUS
100 °F	37 °C
150 °F	65 °C
200 °F	93 °C
250 °F	121 °C
300 °F	150 °C
325 °F	160 °C
350 °F	180 °C
375 °F	190 °C
400 °F	200 °C
425 °F	220 °C
450 °F	230 °C
500 °F	260 °C
525 °F	274 °C
550 °F	288 °C

Weight

IMPERIAL	METRIC
1/2 oz	15 g
1 oz	29 g
2 oz	57 g
3 oz	85 g
4 oz	113 g
5 oz	141 g
6 oz	170 g
8 oz	227 g
10 oz	283 g
12 oz	340 g
13 oz	369 g
14 oz	397 g
15 oz	425 g
1 lb	453 g

Glossary

Acidity Acidity in Extra Virgin Olive Oil refers to the free fatty acid content of the oil. Free fatty acids are formed when fat molecules start to break up.

Alzheimer's disease A form of dementia characterised by a build up of protein "plaques" and "tangles" in the brain.

Anti-inflammatory Something which reduces inflammation. This may describe the property of a chemical or a substance which has the effect.

Antimicrobial This is the ability to be destructive to or inhibiting the growth of microorganisms, including bacteria, viruses, and fungi

Antioxidants These are naturally occurring molecules in our food which can neutralise or mop up free radicals and so repair the damage done through oxidative stress.

Anti-thrombotic This is the effect to reduce the tendency to form blood clots.

Arteriosclerosis The process where fatty deposits and plaques build up on blood vessel walls resulting in diseased, hardened and thickened arteries. This increases the risk of strokes and heart attacks.

Arthritis A term used to describe a range of conditions characterised by pain and inflammation in joints.

Atoms These form part of the make up of all molecules Each atom has a central positively charged core called a nucleus, surrounded by circulating negatively charged pairs of electrons. The pairing of these negatively charged electrons orbiting around the positively charged nucleus makes the atom stable.

Bioactive Compounds These are compounds found in foods providing health benefits beyond basic nutritional requirements and which may reduce pro-inflammatory processes and oxidative stress.

Carbohydrates are made up of sugar and starches. These are known as simple and complex carbohydrates respectively.

Calories This is a measurement of energy in food.

Cancer A disease characterised the abnormal growth of cells resulting in uncontrolled proliferation.

Cardiovascular Relating to the heart or blood vessels.

Carotene A group of fat soluble hydrocarbon orange coloured compounds produced by plants which have been studied for their antioxidant properties.

Cell The smallest structural and functional unit of an organism.

Cholesterol This is a compound found in most body tissues. It has signicant role in the chemistry of our cells. It is also the medium by which chemicals are carried in the blood stream from one part of the body to another. It is made up of high and low density lipids.

Coronary heart disease This describes the condition which is the result of diseased arteries causing a blockage or interruption to the blood supply to the heart.

Dementia The term used to describe a group of symptoms which effect an individual's capacity to think, problem solve, recall events or express themselves.

Deoxyribonucleic acid (DNA) The molecule which carries the genetic instructions for the development, functioning, growth and reproduction of an organism.

Diabetes a condition which causes a person's blood sugar level to be too high. There are different forms of diabetes. It is often associated with other illnesses and diseases.

Electrons Atoms have a central positively charged core called a nucleus, surrounded by circulating negatively charged pairs of electrons.

Embolus A mass of material, usually a blood clot, which causes a blockage to a blood vessel.

Exponential An increasingly rapid rise.

Fats These are made up of different fatty acids joined together along with some non-fatty acid components.

Fatty acids These are complicated molecules consisting of carbon, hydrogen and oxygen atoms bound together with chemical bonds. These chemical bonds may be single or double.

Fibre Plant substances which cannot be fully broken down by the human digestive system. They provide bulk, improve digestive health and have a beneficial effect heart disease, body weight and reduce the risk of some cancers.

Food Matrix This is the nutrient and non-nutrient components of foods and their molecular relationship.

Free Radicals These are unstable by-products of the normal on-going chemical reactions in the body. These products consist of atoms which have lost an electron from a pair. These atoms are unstable and some will "scavenge" electrons from other atoms in the molecules of our cellular structures.

Glyaecemic index/Glyaecemic load The index is a unit measurement representing the effect a particular food has on blood sugar levels. The load is the measured actual effect on blood glucose of the total food or meal consumed.

Glucose A simple sugar, or monosaccharide, which is part of the carbohydrate macronutrient group and which is a source of energy for the body.

Haemorrhage An uncontrolled loss of blood from the circulatory system which can occur as a consequence of rupture of blood vessel wall.

Hexane This is a chemical solvent used in the extraction of oils from seeds or low quality Extra Virgin Olive Oil.

Ibuprofen A widely available drug used to treat inflammation and pain

Immune system This is the structure and processes within our bodies designed to provide defence against disease, including infectious pathogens.

Immunomodulatory This describes the modulation, or regulatory adjustment, of the immune system.

Inflammatory This is the term used to describe the state, where the immune system is involved as part of the body's response to potentially harmful stimuli.

Inflammation can result from external damage or disease and internal chemical processes. Chronic inflammation occurs when the state of inflammation is ongoing and this can be associated with many chronic conditions such as cardiovascular disease, diabetes and cancers.

Insulin A hormone produced by the pancreas which regulates carbohydrates and fats. It acts to ensure safe levels of glucose are maintained and controls the storage and utilisation of energy.

Insulin sensitivity This describes the amount of insulin required by an individual to regulate blood glucose levels. With decreasing sensitivity to the effects of insulin, a person may be said to be increasingly insulin resistant.

Legumes A type of plant, for example beans or peas, with edible seeds that grow in cases, or pods. The pods themselves are often edible also.

Lignans A group of plant chemicals belonging to the polyphenol class which have antioxidant properties.

Meta analyses This is the joint analysis of the several published studies to analyse the combined results.

Metabolic The chemical processes which occur in cells of organisms which are necessary for the maintenance of life.

Micronutrients The life sustaining components in foods which are generally required in relatively small amounts but which may have a very significant effect on health.

Molecules All of the structures in our bodies are made up of molecules which consist of atoms joined together in particular patterns.

Monounsaturated fatty acid These have a chemical structure with only one double bond in their entire structure.

Neuroprotective This is the capacity to protect nerve cells against damage, degeneration, or impairment of function.

Nutrients The components in foods which sustain life.

Obesity This describes a state of being grossly overweight, and is associated with increased risks of illness and disease.

Oleic acid This is a monounsaturated fatty acid. It is the predominant fat in Extra Virgin Olive Oil and derives its name from the olive.

Oleocanthal This is a specific polyphenol found in Extra Virgin Olive Oil which has antioxidant and anti-inflammatory properties.

Omega 3 fatty acid This is a polyunsaturated fatty acid which the body is unable to manufacture or itself. It has bonds in the third position of the fatty acid molecule. The most common Omega 3 fatty acid is also known as alphalinolenic acid.

Omega 6 fatty acid This is a polyunsaturated fatty acid which the body is unable to manufacture for itself. It has bonds are in the sixth position of the fatty acid molecule. The most common Omega 6 fat is called linoleic acid.

Omega 9 This is a monounsaturated fatty acid which the body is unable to manufacture for itself. It has bond in the ninth position of the fatty acid molecule. The most common Omega 9 is also known as Oleic acid.

Osteoarthritis A condition characterised by painful and stiff joints, which may become swollen and cause disability.

Oxidation This is when an atom or molecule loses one or more electrons in a chemical reaction.

Oxidative stress This occurs when free radicals attack and damage cells in the body through oxidation. This has pro-inflammatory effects.

Palmitic acid This is a saturated fatty acid which is thought to be one of the most harmful.

Parkinson's disease A condition where a part of the brain becomes progressively damaged, having an effect particularly on movement, though which may also result in decline in memory, language and more general psychological and physical effects.

Pathogen This is any small organism, such as a virus or a bacterium that can cause disease.

Peroxide These are chemicals that are formed when fats break down as result of oxidation.

Phenol This is a molecule of hydrogen and oxygen with a hexagonal structure. Some of the most complex chemicals found in our foods are made up of lots of phenols in various different combinations, therefore called polyphenols. Tyrosol, found in Extra Virgin Olive Oil is a good example.

Phenolic See Phenols.

Phyto-nutrients Vitamins, minerals and anitoxidants carried in the coloured pigments of many plants. Also known as Phyto-chemicals.

Plaques Plaque formation on the inner surface of blood vessel walls is part of a complex process involved in arteriosclerosis, eventually resulting in diseased arteries.

Platelets Blood cells, the function of which is to promote the formation of clots. This is primarily designed to prevent haemorrhage when blood vessel walls are damaged.

Polyphenols See Phenols.

Polyunsaturated fatty acid These have a chemical structure with more than one double bond between the carbon atoms.

Pomace This is the name given to the residue of olive flesh and stones that remains after the oil has been extracted.

Pro-inflammatory A process or state resulting in increased inflammation.

Pulses Members of the legume family of plants, the edible seeds of which are often dried as foods.

Rancidity the effect of decomposition, especially of edible fats through oxidation, resulting in a foul taste and smell.

Redox This is the name given to a balanced state of equilibrium in cells where any oxidative stress is balanced by our cells natural antioxidant capacity.

Rheumatoid Arthritis An autoimmune disease of joints characterised by inflammation, pain, swelling and stiffness especially, though not exclusively involving the joints of the hands and feet.

Saturated fatty acids These have a chemical structure with no double bonds in their make up. All the carbon atoms are linked to hydrogen atoms.

Spectrophotometer This is a machine which measures the absorption of UV light at specific wavelengths to detect levels of particular chemical/molecules. It relies on the principle that certain compounds have particular patterns of absorption or transmission of UV light.

Squalene A specific hydrocarbon molecule found in the body and also in certain foods which has been the subject of research for its possible anti cancer effects.

Telomeres These are protective caps on the stands of DNA which makes up our chromosomes. They get shorter every time a cell divides.

Transfats These are unsaturated fats which have undergone "hydrogenation". This is chemical process in which hydrogen is added to the original fat molecule.

Tri-glycerides A fat which is comprised of three fatty acids attached to a molecule called glycerol.

Ulcerative Colitis This is a disease where bowel symptoms occur as a consequence of inflammation of the wall of the colon - the lower part of the gastrointestinal tract.

Vitamins These are essential micronutrients which are needed for health and which the body is unable to manufacture for itself.

Index